Jeffrey T. Huber, PhD

HIV/AIDS Community Information Services: Experiences in Serving Both At-Risk and Hiv-Infected Populations

Pre-publication REVIEWS, COMMENTARIES, EVALUATIONS . . .

"Information is the first step in the acquisition of knowledge and forms the basis for all education, which is currently the primary means to prevent the spread of HIV infection. However, information access to the vast array of resources available in both traditional and nontraditional formats can be confusing and intimidating. Huber's book provides a well-organized introduction to the provision of information services that will be useful to those affected by HIV disease, health care practitioners, librarians, and other information professionals. He examines resources presently available, including library programs focusing on HIV/AIDS, specialized information centers, AIDS-specific electronic sources, and information networks between AIDS service organizations, community-based organizations, and national organizations. The material on electronic resources, including the Internet, will be particularly useful to readers with limited knowledge of computer technologies. This book is an excellent introductory resource to guide the reader to the acquisition of HIV/AIDS information."

J. Michael Howe, MSLS
Manager/Biological and Medical Sciences Librarian, Department of Veterans Affairs AIDS Information Center, VA Medical Center, San Francisco, CA

More pre-publication
REVIEWS, COMMENTARIES, EVALUATIONS . . .

"In *HIV/AIDS Community Information Services*, Dr. Jeffrey Huber clearly and concisely articulates what many of us in the AIDS information dissemination arena have been wrestling with for years. How can we as health information professionals effectively identify, evaluate, and disseminate information about HIV/AIDS and at the same time promote knowledge acquisition in order to prevent the spread of this pandemic? Huber's contribution establishes a paradigm for understanding how HIV/AIDS information is created and consumed, labels the forces at play and focuses us on the key tasks at hand. He reminds us that education is the only hold that will pin HIV/AIDS to the mat until a cure or vaccine is found.

Early in the book, Huber relates the need to translate information into knowledge in order to effectively deal with HIV/AIDS. He then addresses the many social, political, religious, and cultural intricacies that have proved handicaps in effectively translating HIV/AIDS information into the knowledge that will save lives. His discussion of the implications of using an epidemiologically derived case definition of HIV/AIDS in particular sheds much-needed light on the complexities of serving our many HIV/AIDS information constituencies.

Huber reminds readers of the nontraditional models of HIV/AIDS information creation and dissemination, often in the forms of newsletters, usenet news groups, and community-based service publications. He surveys the key electronic bibliographic and full-text resources available, and describes current proactive partnerships between HIV/AIDS information producers and consumers. The Appendixes include a list of networked electronic resources, a complete discussion of the case definition of HIV/AIDS, and a brief but targeted list of relevant organizations. The book is easy to use and logical in organization and progression.

HIV/AIDS Community Information Services is balm for the bruised and weary. It provides a construct for understanding why it has been so hard to provide effective HIV/AIDS information services. Huber's work simultaneously exhorts us, especially in light of the proliferation of electronic resources available via the Internet, to take a proactive stance as we continue to rally to the HIV/AIDS information cause."

Gerald J. Perry, MLS
Reference Manager and
Collection Development Specialist,
Library of Rush University,
Chicago, IL

NOTES FOR PROFESSIONAL LIBRARIANS AND LIBRARY USERS

This is an original book title published by The Haworth Press, Inc. Unless otherwise noted in specific chapters with attribution, materials in this book have not been previously published elsewhere in any format or language.

CONSERVATION AND PRESERVATION NOTES

All books published by The Haworth Press, Inc. and its imprints are printed on certified ph neutral, acid free book grade paper. This paper meets the minimum requirements of American National Standard for Information Sciences–Permanence of Paper for Printed Material, ANSI Z39.48-1984.

HIV/AIDS Community Information Services
Experiences in Serving Both At-Risk and HIV-Infected Populations

HAWORTH Medical Information Sources
M. Sandra Wood, MLS, MBA
Senior Editor

New, Recent, and Forthcoming Titles:

How to Find Information About AIDS, 2nd Edition edited by Jeffrey T. Huber

CD-ROM Implementation and Networking in Health Sciences Libraries edited by M. Sandra Wood

User Education in Health Sciences Libraries: A Reader edited by M. Sandra Wood

HIV/AIDS Community Information Services: Experiences in Serving Both At-Risk and HIV-Infected Populations by Jeffrey T. Huber

HIV/AIDS and HIV/AIDS-Related Terminology: A Means of Organizing the Body of Knowledge by Jeffrey T. Huber and Mary L. Gillaspy

HIV/AIDS Community Information Services

Experiences in Serving Both At-Risk and HIV-Infected Populations

Jeffrey T. Huber, PhD

The Haworth Press
New York • London

The Haworth Press, Inc., 10 Alice Street, Binghamton, NY 13904-1580

Library of Congress Cataloging-in-Publication Data

Huber, Jeffrey T.
HIV/AIDS community information services : experiences in serving both at-risk and HIV-infected populations / Jeffrey T. Huber.
p. cm.
Includes bibliographical references and index.
ISBN 1-56024-940-4 (alk. paper)
1. AIDS (Disease)–Information services. 2. Community health services. I. Title.
RA644.A25H83 1996
362.1'969792–dc20 95-51653
CIP

For Robert

A closed door,
and an open window.

ABOUT THE AUTHOR

Jeffrey T. Huber, PhD, is currently Research Information Scientist at Vanderbilt University in Nashville, Tennessee. Until recently, he was Assistant Professor at the School of Library and Information Studies at Texas Women's University in Denton, Texas, where he was also Co-Chair of the University's Task Force on HIV/AIDS. Dr. Huber is the author of a number of articles concerning AIDS information and is the editor of *How to Find Information About AIDS, Second Edition* and *Dictionary of AIDS-Related Terminology*. A member of the American Library Association, the Medical Library Association, and the International Society for AIDS Education, Dr. Huber has delivered many presentations at national conferences and meetings.

CONTENTS

Introduction

The human immunodeficiency virus (HIV) and the acquired immunodeficiency syndrome (AIDS) have created a modern health care dilemma that pervades the world community. No industry–including those concerned with the creation, evaluation, organization, storage, retrieval, and dissemination of information–remains unaffected. If one examines the paradigm of information-knowledge-wisdom, information forms the first step in the acquisition of knowledge and possible subsequent conversion of that knowledge into wisdom. Information may be equated with data, facts, or figures; knowledge connotes understanding; and wisdom implies insight. The progression along the continuum, however, is dependent upon the initial provision of information. This model functions as the foundation for the education process. Information forms the basis for all education, and currently education is the only weapon available to stem the spread of the AIDS epidemic and foster empathy toward those individuals already affected by this disease. In addition, information continues to serve as a source of recreation and entertainment to HIV-infected individuals.

While directories currently exist to assist with practical approaches in accessing HIV/AIDS-related information, there is no resource concerning the nature of that information or the provision of information services. This work is designed to fill that void. The purpose of this book is to facilitate the provision of information services–both educational and recreational–to individuals infected with the human immunodeficiency virus and to promote the dissemination of instructional materials to those individuals who are at risk for infection. Through the provision of information, it is also hoped that this work will serve as a tool to foster the enlightenment of the general public concerning the true nature of this illness. As a greater portion of the HIV-infected population progresses to the development of AIDS, information will be in greater demand and increasingly difficult to provide.

This book is organized in a logical sequence designed to provide the reader with an understanding of the information construct within the AIDS arena and how that construct influences the provision of information to an HIV-affected population. Chapter 1 presents an overview of the complicated nature of the HIV/AIDS pandemic. Included is a discussion of the legal, medical, psychological, religious, and social complexities commonly associated with the disease. This overview establishes the connection between HIV/AIDS and the body of information concerning the epidemic, and lays the foundation for examining the complex nature of AIDS-related data. Having established the construct under which HIV/AIDS information exists, Chapter 2 examines the types of information currently available including a cursory discussion of sources and resources for accessing these materials. It also describes some of the barriers to accessing AIDS-related information such as nontraditional publication channels, collection development and acquisition practices, and cataloging and indexing policies. Chapter 3 examines more closely specialized information resources presently available. This discussion includes such things as existing library programs focusing on HIV/AIDS, specialized information centers such as the National AIDS Clearinghouse, ready reference sources such as the National AIDS Hotline, and AIDS-specific electronic sources of information such as those available through the National Library of Medicine (e.g., AIDSLINE, AIDSTRIALS, and AIDSDRUGS). Non-U.S. (foreign) examples are included whenever possible. Chapter 4 focuses on HIV/AIDS information resource sharing. This chapter examines existing information networks between AIDS service organizations, community-based organizations, information clearinghouses, libraries, national organizations, and international organizations. Chapter 5 explores potential areas for future development to enhance and expand existing information services in order to better serve the HIV-affected population. Following Chapter 5 is a series of appendixes: Appendix A contains the case definitions of AIDS; Appendix B contains AIDS classification systems; Appendix C contains sample Internet resources; and Appendix D contains directory information for organizations and institutions referred to in the text.

This book is not designed to serve as a comprehensive HIV/AIDS information resource but examines a theoretical approach to the nature of the information and the provision of services, with practical examples throughout for illustration. It is bound by the same limitations that are discussed within each chapter. The work is presented as a guide to foster the creation, accession, collection, organization, dissemination, and sharing of information concerning the HIV/AIDS epidemic; and to encourage the provision of services to individuals affected by the human immunodeficiency virus and the acquired immunodeficiency syndrome.

Chapter 1

The Complex Nature of the Epidemic

THE HUMAN IMMUNODEFICIENCY VIRUS AND THE ACQUIRED IMMUNODEFICIENCY SYNDROME: A STUDY IN CONTROVERSIES AND COMPLEXITIES

Although the acquired immunodeficiency syndrome is clearly defined in biomedical terms and for the biomedical community, an AIDS diagnosis reaches far beyond biomedicine. The impact of this disease calls for a multidisciplinary response. With the abundant growth in the prevalence of AIDS cases, each additional diagnosis–wittingly or otherwise–ripples through the local community to society at large. The social construct within which HIV and AIDS exist cannot be ignored.

THE NATURE, SCOPE, AND COMPLEXITIES OF DEFINING HIV/AIDS

The Treatment of HIV Infection as a Disease

At the outset, the illness that we now call AIDS (the nomenclature assigned in the summer of 1982) was known by a host of names including, but not limited to, GRID (gay-related immune deficiency), ACIDS (acquired community immune deficiency syndrome), and CAIDS (community acquired immune deficiency syndrome).

In order to understand better the complex nature of this illness, it is necessary to examine the treatment of HIV infection as a disease. Spatialization of disease has been plotted by Foucault in an historical continuum that parallels the development of the scientific foundation for modern medicine (anatomical pathology) and societal delineation of the pathological. This spatialization of the pathological has been characterized as (1) primary (configuration of the disease); (2) secondary (localization of the illness in the body); (3) tertiary (ordered and presented in a manner deemed suitable by and to society); and (4) quaternary (institutional spatialization of the illness).[1] In the context of HIV and AIDS, however, this historical continuum disintegrates, and spatialization digresses to its primitive form while remaining socially circumscribed.

Primary spatialization of the pathological is concerned with the nosological picture of the disease—how the illness is described or classified. This classificatory theory does not account for the causes and effects of the illness, the constellation of signs and symptoms that accumulate to form a chronological series of events, or the visible trajectory of the malady within the human body. In the case of HIV infection and AIDS, this initial spatialization may be evinced in the nomenclature first used to describe the disease—the gay plague, gay bowel syndrome, gay-related immune deficiency. In classifying the illness at the outset of the epidemic, terminology was employed assigning the pathological to the population initially thought to be most affected rather than describing the malady itself. The terminology used was designed to define an unknown fear. In this manner, the individual affected by HIV/AIDS received no positive status. Thus, the politicization and stigmatization that continue to circumscribe the pandemic were established.

In secondary spatialization of disease, the illness is mapped out upon the concrete structure of the human body. This articulation of the pathological on the body requires knowledge of basic anatomy that can be obtained only through the physical examination of the diseased tissue. The patient becomes essential to identifying and understanding the clearly ordered forms of the malady. Initially however, the acceptance of dissection–the foundation for pathological anatomy–faced several obstacles including, but not limited to, morality, religion, and prejudice. Once a positive observation of dissection for the purpose of studying and understanding diseased tissue and its relation to the various parts of the body was established, "the knowledge of the living, ambiguous disease could be aligned upon the white visibility of the dead."[2]

The problem with the secondary spatialization of HIV/AIDS, in part, is that the politicization and stigmatization established under primary delineation has not been overcome. Obstacles once barring the introduction and use of dissection–such as morality, religion, and prejudice–continue to be associated with this disease. Many individuals with HIV remain unidentified, both in life and in death. This anonymity is often achieved and upheld through a desire on the part of the individual affected by the illness not to be identified as an HIV-infected body. The pandemic has forced renewed examination of culturally sensitive subjects–death, homosexuality, human sexuality–that society has historically chosen to censor or ignore. While these issues commonly associated with the epidemic are in fact a very real part of life, the ramifications of owning an HIV diagnosis or developing AIDS are multiple and often overwhelming. In addition, many physicians do not wish to work with HIV-infected bodies. Where a close proximity between patient and physician is required in order to progress to a true secondary spatialization of HIV/AIDS, all too often a wedge has been driven between these two necessary factions preventing the examination of the infected tissue.

Tertiary spatialization of the pathological is defined in terms of social space–societal regimens and upheavals, economic constraints, political ambitions, utopian ideas–confronting both primary and secondary identifications of disease. The structure of these two factions (social versus medical) are of very different natures, as are the laws governing each body. The result of this confrontation is illness presented in terms of "all gestures by which, in a given society, a disease is circumscribed, medically invested, isolated, divided up into closed, privileged regions, or distributed throughout cure centres, arranged in the most favorable way."[3] Society takes what is medically proven and represents it in a manner found to be acceptable, not offensive. For HIV/AIDS, this tertiary spatialization exacerbates the politicization and stigmatization established under its primary description, and further complicates the problems evinced in its secondary delineation. The disease, when and if it is discussed, becomes surrounded by a host of metaphors, euphemisms, and misinformation rather than accurate terminology. In an extreme effort not to offend society, quarantine and isolation become very real possibilities. Laws are sought to protect society from those infected. For the person with HIV, this social spatialization may be likened to abandonment, ostracism, or banishment.

The final step in the continuum of the development of modern medicine (or the quaternary spatialization of disease) consists of the institutionalization of the pathological. "The medicine of spaces disappears."[4] Primary, secondary, and tertiary spatialization of illness mesh together, resulting in a medicine that is invested with a genesis, power, rationality, and structure of its own. The goals of society and medicine combine, ensuring that the art of curing continues to exist and flourish. HIV/AIDS, unlike most diseases, has not yet reached this plateau. The many legal, medical, psychological, religious, and social complexities that riddle its space have prevented this from being the case. In essence, the human immunodeficiency virus and the acquired immunodeficiency syndrome continue to be defined and circumscribed by primitive spatialization, to exist in a medicine of spaces rather than on an integral plane that fosters empathy and compassion.

Defining HIV/AIDS

In 1981, shortly after the first cases were diagnosed, the Centers for Disease Control (CDC)–now the Centers for Disease Control and Prevention–established a surveillance case definition in an effort to monitor the spread of the disease. However, it was limited in that the definition detailed a prescribed list of opportunistic infections that had to meet specific criteria for definitive, as opposed to presumptive, diagnosis.

In subsequent years–as more began to be known and understood about the disease–the need for a definition which allowed for more sensitivity in case assessment became apparent. So, in 1985 the prior CDC surveillance case definition was expanded to include such pathogenic conditions as certain non-Hodgkin's lymphomas, chronic isosporiasis, and disseminated histoplasmosis.[5]

By 1987, it had become evident that the 1985 revision of the case definition was inadequate; so the Centers for Disease Control issued the "Revision of the CDC Surveillance Case Definition for Acquired Immunodeficiency Syndrome."[6] The objectives of the amended version included: (1) to track more effectively the severe morbidity associated with HIV infection; (2) to simplify reporting of AIDS cases; (3) to increase the sensitivity and specificity through the application of HIV-antibody laboratory tests; and (4) to be consistent with current diagnostic practices. This final clause allowed for inclusion based on presumptive–rather than definitive–diagnosis for several diseases such as *Pneumocystis carinii* pneumonia (PCP), Kaposi's sarcoma (KS), and toxoplasmosis of the brain. The revised definition also included the addition of several definitively diagnosed diseases when accompanied by laboratory evidence for HIV infection such as HIV encephalopathy (HIV dementia), HIV wasting syndrome (slim disease, cachexia), and extrapulmonary tuberculosis; thereby expanding the field of indicator diseases to encompass a more diverse collection of clinical manifestations.[7]

It should be noted that the CDC definition was developed for epidemiologic surveillance, and not as a description of the disease. This has direct impact on the degree of AIDS-related assistance for which an individual may qualify, since the CDC definition typically serves as the determinant for AIDS-related policies and procedures. The revised definition neither comprised every HIV-related illness, nor did it account for all causes of morbidity resulting from HIV.[8] Similarly, the revision did not include any specific gynecological indications of HIV infection.

In an effort to more accurately reflect the manifestations of HIV and those individuals infected with the virus, the CDC revised the definition again in 1993. The major additions under this revision included: (1) the inclusion of three clinical conditions–pulmonary tuberculosis, recurrent pneumonia, and invasive cervical cancer; and (2) all HIV-infected persons who have a CD4+ T-lymphocyte count less than 200 cells per cubic millimeter of blood. Although the indicative criteria for reporting cases of AIDS has, to date, been revised three times, it is probable that the definition will continue to evolve–thus reflecting the increased understanding of the pandemic. (See Appendix A for various manifestations of the case definition of AIDS.)

As was the case with the acronym *AIDS,* the term *HIV* developed over the course of the epidemic and was preceded by other names. Luc Montagnier dubbed the retrovirus (discovered by him and his research team in 1983 at the Pasteur Institute) lymphadenopathy-associated virus (LAV). Shortly after Montagnier's discovery, Robert Gallo at the National Institutes of Health declared the retrovirus he discovered in 1984 to be human T-cell lymphotropic virus III (HTLV-III). After much controversy, it was learned that the two discoveries were, in fact, the same. Therefore, the retrovirus was renamed as the human immunodeficiency virus (HIV) and it is this virus that is believed to cause

AIDS. This final christening, however, did not ensure the immediate replacement of previously accepted terms.

HIV and AIDS, although not synonymous, are often used interchangeably. According to the surveillance case definition, infection with the human immunodeficiency virus has direct implications for an AIDS diagnosis. However, it is not uncommon for the term *AIDS virus* to be used rather than HIV. In point of fact, HIV refers to the virus that suppresses the human immune system, thus promoting various opportunistic infections and/or cancers which produce a constellation of symptoms known as the acquired immunodeficiency syndrome. Someone who is HIV infected does not necessarily have AIDS.

In the model progression of HIV and AIDS, an individual is first infected with the human immunodeficiency virus and subsequently is diagnosed with the acquired immunodeficiency syndrome. However, in reality, this is not always the case. Many individuals first discover they have been HIV infected at the time of their AIDS diagnoses. Some individuals, while aware of being infected, may progress quickly to full-blown AIDS while others may be long-term survivors or nonprogressors (individuals who are HIV infected but show no decline in CD4 counts over a period of seven to 12 years). This is further complicated by a lack of consistency, and lack of precision, in use of the terminology. As stated previously, being diagnosed HIV positive does not constitute having developed AIDS–a distinction critical within the AIDS arena but continuously overlooked. Conversely, as the definition of AIDS continues to evolve and grow (reflecting the recognized changes within the epidemic and encompassing more sensitive diagnostic procedures), the distinctions concerning disease progression will be blurred.

Under the current surveillance case definition, only those individuals manifesting clinical and laboratory manifestations which meet the CDC criteria qualify for an AIDS diagnosis. Since many illnesses associated with HIV are common in persons who are not infected with the human immunodeficiency virus, exclusions of HIV-related conditions are not uncommon.

The implications of accepting, and adhering to, the current definition of AIDS are manifold. Since the CDC definition was developed for epidemiologic surveillance purposes, it cannot be construed as a description of all clinical presentations of the disease. Conditions exist which, although falling within the spectrum of HIV-related clinical manifestations, are not reflected in the surveillance case definition. Thus, certain conditions based on the CDC definition and related to HIV are not considered in AIDS-related policies, procedures, and legislation. Similarly, reporting standards are generally based on cases of full-blown AIDS, and not positive HIV diagnoses. This allows statistics to be skewed since the estimated number of individuals infected with the human immunodeficiency virus far outweighs the number of reported cases of AIDS. It should also be noted that, due in part to the stigma associated with the disease, reported statistics are, at best, understated. In addition, the medical complexities of the disease further complicate the application of the definition.

The 1993 Revised CDC Surveillance Case Definition

The 1993 revision of the CDC surveillance case definition includes all HIV-infected persons with CD4+ T-lymphocyte counts of less than 200 cells per cubic millimeter of blood or a CD4+ percentage of less than 14. In addition, the following clinical conditions serve as diagnostic criteria for AIDS-defining conditions: (1) candidiasis of the bronchi, trachea, or lungs; (2) candidiasis of the esophagus; (3) invasive cervical cancer; (4) disseminated or extrapulmonary coccidioidomycosis; (5) extrapulmonary cryptococcosis; (6) chronic intestinal cryptosporidiosis (more than one month's duration); (7) cytomegalovirus disease (other than liver, spleen, or nodes); (8) cytomegalovirus retinitis (with loss of vision); (9) HIV-related encephalopathy; (10) herpes simplex: chronic ulcer(s) (more than one month's duration); or bronchitis, pneumonitis, or esophagitis; (11) disseminated or extrapulmonary histoplasmosis; (12) chronic intestinal isosporiasis (more than one month's duration); (13) Kaposi's sarcoma; (14) Burkitt's lymphoma (or equivalent term); (15) immunoblastic lymphoma (or equivalent term); (16) primary lymphoma of the brain; (17) disseminated or extrapulmonary Mycobacterium avium complex or Mycobacterium kansasii; (18) pulmonary or extrapulmonary Mycobacterium tuberculosis; (19) disseminated or extrapulmonary Mycobacterium other species; (20) *Pneumocystis carinii* pneumonia; (21) recurrent pneumonia; (22) progressive multifocal leukoencephalopathy; (23) recurrent salmonella septicemia; (24) toxoplasmosis of the brain; or (25) wasting syndrome due to HIV.[9]

AIDS EPIDEMIOLOGY

Epidemiology may be defined as that branch of medicine which deals with defining and explaining the interrelationships of the factors determining disease frequency and distribution. For AIDS, the criteria on which the reporting standards are based is the CDC surveillance case definition. Although two strains of HIV have been isolated (HIV-1 and HIV-2), reports are generally limited to HIV-1 "as virtually no epidemiologic or natural history data on HIV type 2 exist."[10] HIV-2 has proven, thus far, to be more common in West Africa, although a few cases have been documented in the United States.

Modes of HIV Transmission

While traces of HIV have been found in saliva, sweat, and tears, it is generally accepted that the exchange of these bodily fluids is not an efficient mode of transmission. The risk of becoming HIV infected through blood transfusions has largely been eliminated in the United States due to the strict screening processes implemented for all blood donations. There has been some recent concern, however, regarding transplants using donated organs, as the donor may have been so recently infected that there has not been ample time for seroconversion (the change in a test result from negative to positive for the presence of antibodies in response to HIV infection) and the donated organs test negative rather than positive. Health care and laboratory personnel are at a limited risk if they work with infected instruments, blood, or tissue samples. Health care facilities have attempted to alleviate this risk by adopting universal precautions to minimize exposure to blood and other body fluids and tissues. HIV continues to be efficiently spread, however, through unprotected sexual intercourse, the sharing of needles and/or syringes, and perinatally from mother to fetus. While the majority of reported AIDS cases are attributed to a single mode of exposure, approximately 13 percent are ascribed to multiple modes of exposure–there are homosexual/bisexual men who use IV drugs, just as there are IV drug users who have sex with heterosexuals who have been exposed to HIV.[11]

Unprotected sexual intercourse places both parties involved at risk for infection. HIV has been isolated from both semen and vaginal secretions. Anal intercourse–especially among men–is an acutely effective mode of HIV transmission. Men who have sex with men continue to comprise the greatest number of reported AIDS cases in the United States, with more than 60 percent of the total attributed to exposure to male homosexual/bisexual contact.[12] (The United States, however, is the only country where men who have sex with men comprise the largest population who are HIV infected or who have AIDS.) Receptive (passive) anal intercourse is markedly more risky than insertive (active). Moreover, oral sex–which originally was thought to pose no threat for infection–serves as a somewhat less efficient mode of transmission, but a mode nonetheless with a few reported cases having ascribed infection to this path. Vaginal intercourse also serves as an efficient means for transmitting the virus. Male-to-female transmission–as with insertive rather than receptive anal intercourse–is more effective than female-to-male, but both modes of exposure are sufficiently documented. This is especially true in countries where the vast majority of cases involve heterosexual transmission, such as in Africa or the Caribbean islands.[13] In the United States, heterosexual contact accounts for approximately 7 percent of the total reported cases.[14]

Intravenous drug users (IVDUs) comprise the second largest at-risk population in the United States, with approximately 25 percent of the total reported cases of AIDS being credited to the injecting drug use exposure category.[15] With this mode of HIV transmission, the two dominant risk factors are the frequency of injections and the use of shared works (paraphernalia necessary for injection such as needles and syringes).[16] Each incidence of injecting drugs increases the potential for exposure to HIV. Contaminated needles or syringes, which are tainted with infected blood, effectively transport the virus and provide the means for bodily invasion upon insertion into the vein. Booting–the practice of withdrawing blood into the narcotic-filled syringe prior to injecting the entire contents for the purpose of enhancing the drug-induced high–increases the risk for transmission by furthering exposure to the virus.

Mothers who are HIV infected transmit the virus to approximately 30 percent of their babies.[17] Of AIDS cases involving children under the age of 13 which have been reported to the CDC, approximately 89 percent are attributed to HIV-infected mothers.[18] In perinatal transmission, it is not certain whether the virus infects the fetus through the placenta, during placental separation when fetal and maternal blood mix, during movement through the birth canal when the fetus is exposed to mucosal contact or may ingest bodily fluids, or by a combination of these. Additionally, the virus has been isolated in breast milk, but this has been documented as a mode of transmission with uncertain efficiency as there are few recorded examples.

It is important to note that it is the behavior that places an individual at risk for infection, not belonging to a particular group or population. Because someone is gay does not mean that he or she is likely to be infected with HIV. A female engaging in unprotected sexual intercourse places herself at risk for infection as does a male practicing unsafe sex.

Cofactors of HIV Infection and Progression

In spite of the fact that AIDS does not discriminate (by race, religious beliefs, socioeconomic background, or sexual orientation), there are certain cofactors which may increase the risk for HIV infection or advance the course of the illness. With the exception of age, however, the influence of cofactors continues to be debated. Diseases which result in genital ulcers, such as chancroid, augment the risk for HIV infection. Genital ulcers that are less severe in nature, such as those associated with primary syphilis, also facilitate transmission of the virus. The very nature of the lesions exacerbates the risk and multiplies the possibilities for successful viral contact. Similarly, uncircumcised men have been shown to be at greater risk for infection than circumcised, as the foreskin provides a suitable habitat to prolong exposure to the virus.

Although uncertain as to the extent of its contribution, coinfections with other viruses are believed to influence the progression of the human immunodeficiency virus. "It has long been suspected that AIDS incidence might be affected by a subtle interplay between viral and host factors."[19] Moreover, certain strains of HIV appear to be more virulent than others; thus the strain of infection may help to determine the course of the disease. Stress is also generally accepted to negatively affect the human immune system, which in turn may contribute to HIV progression.

Even though the role that cofactors play in the transmission and progression of HIV is not completely understood, the fact remains that the median time of progression from infection with the human immunodeficiency virus to the development of full-blown AIDS for adults is seven to ten years. Although not every HIV-infected individual progresses to the onset of AIDS–some continue to remain asymptomatic, others present with clinical manifestations that do not qualify for an AIDS diagnosis–the majority manifest the signs and symptoms of the illness over a period of time. There are those, however, who die without meeting the criteria established by the definition. It is imperative to note that the CDC surveillance case definition consists of a list of predefined conditions and diseases that are not necessarily representative of all manifestations or complications of HIV. However, it has been estimated that 50 percent of those infected will develop CDC-defined AIDS within ten to 11 years of their initial infection.[20] "On the whole, it appears today that the most important predictors of progression from HIV infection to AIDS are the symptom complex (if any) at the time the person learns of his infection and the length of time an individual has been infected."[21]

HIV Classification Schemes

At least two classification schemes have been proposed to gauge the degree of infection with the human immunodeficiency virus. Both staging systems were developed in an effort to more effectively represent HIV infection, as opposed to strictly adhering to the CDC surveillance case definition for AIDS. The system initially put forth by the CDC was based on clinical manifestations, and was divided into four groups designated by Roman numerals. Group I included HIV-infected individuals who had seroconverted and presented with a mononucleosis-like syndrome. Group II included individuals who had tested HIV positive but were asymptomatic. Group III included those individuals with persistent generalized lymphadenopathy (PGL), but no other symptoms. Group IV included all symptomatic HIV-infected individuals, and was subdivided by disease manifestation.[22] The system proposed by the Walter Reed Army Institute of Research classifies the stages of infection with the human immunodeficiency virus according to the presence or absence of T helper cells, chronic lymphadenopathy, delayed hypersensitivity, thrush, and opportunistic infections. This system is applicable only to adults, as the baseline functional T-cell index on which the scale is based may vary in neonates, infants, and children. The classification scheme is divided into seven categories with appropriate subcategories. These are designated WR0 to WR6, with subcategories being represented by the addition of alphabetical abbreviations–K for Kaposi's sarcoma, N for neoplasms other than Kaposi's sarcoma, or CNS for central nervous system.[23] However, both systems have been criticized as being unsatisfactory.

In the "1993 Revised Classification System for HIV Infection and Expanded Case Surveillance Case Definition for AIDS Among Adolescents and Adults," the CDC revised their classification system to categorize persons on the basis of clinical conditions associated with HIV infection and CD4+ T-lymphocyte counts. The system is based on three ranges of CD4+ T-lymphocyte counts and three clinical categories, and is represented by a matrix of nine mutually exclusive categories. This system replaces the classification system published in 1986, which included only clinical disease criteria and which was developed before the widespread use of CD4+ T-cell testing.[24] (See Appendix B for the various classification systems.)

HIV AND AIDS: THE LEGAL, MEDICAL, AND PSYCHOSOCIAL ISSUES

Multifarious, interrelated, complex issues comprise the web which further complicates a positive HIV-antibody test result, or medical diagnosis of AIDS. These issues, in addition to the clinical manifestations, may have direct impact on all involved.

Legal

To date there is no other single infectious disease in the history of the American legal system that has generated more litigation than the human immunodeficiency virus.[25] Three issues have been central to the legal and ethical concerns regarding the acquired immunodeficiency syndrome: discrimination against HIV-infected individuals, confidentiality and its boundaries, and the exercise of compulsory government powers to stem the spread of the epidemic.[26] Discrimination, in most instances, is founded on an irrational fear of AIDS. These fears include such apprehensions as homophobia, contagion, and death. Discrimination has been evinced in the exclusion of HIV-infected adults and children from educational facilities, insurance, housing, and jobs. All too often, these fears have mushroomed to the point of hostility. This is especially true among certain populations often perceived to be at risk–gay men in particular. Although considered a handicap and protected under antidiscriminatory legislation (the Federal Rehabilitation Act of 1973 and similar handicap statutes at the state level), the infected continue to bear the brunt of AIDS-related discrimination, although at this writing the discrimination is more covert than before.

Confidentiality remains an ongoing debate. The controversy includes such issues as reporting by name those persons who have a positive HIV test result (including those who are asymptomatic); breaching the physician/patient trust in order to promote contact tracing for the purpose of warning third parties at risk; maintaining records based on reporting of HIV test results and/or contact tracing; and designating by name those individuals who have AIDS, are HIV positive, or practice high risk behaviors. Contact tracing has been at issue since it has the potential to facilitate the creation and maintenance of a registry of names–names self-reported by individuals who receive the test for the presence of the HIV antibody, whether positive or negative–that may be used in some way to "control" the spread of the epidemic. Confidentiality continues to be of paramount concern in the AIDS arena due, in large part, to the stigmatization associated with the illness.

Government coercion to stem the spread of the disease has met with a great deal of opposition. The coercion involves mandatory testing for the presence of the HIV antibody, isolation or quarantine (in the event of positive test results or an AIDS diagnosis), applying criminal litigation practices and procedures to the intentional transmission of the human immunodeficiency virus, and creating and implementing public health statutes that are AIDS-specific. The difficulties in applying any of these compulsory means to limit the spread of the epidemic, quite obviously, rests in weighing (on the scales of human justice) the difference between individual rights and public health.

Neither a cure for AIDS nor a vaccine to prevent HIV infection–it is generally agreed–is in the near future. "On a more positive note, however, gradual and less dramatic advances have helped to increase understanding of the pathophysiology of the infection, to delay the onset of physical symptoms, and to treat opportunistic infections and tumors when they arise."[27] Unfortunately, the case-fatality rate continues to be in excess of 60 percent.[28]

Medical

The human immunodeficiency virus–HIV-1 and HIV-2 are genetically related, with HIV-2 considered to be less virulent–is a parasite which is dependent upon host cells for survival. This is why it cannot be transmitted via an inanimate object, such as a toilet seat. The human immunodeficiency virus is a retrovirus; and like other retroviruses, it consists of ribonucleic acid (RNA) and lacks deoxyribonucleic acid (DNA), and cannot replicate in the usual way. It carries reverse transcriptase, or an enzyme which catalyzes the process of forming a compound (by combining simpler molecules) in order to synthesize DNA using certain aspects of RNA. The DNA copy is then incorporated into the chromosomes of the host cell, which is thereby programmed with the viral genetic code. When the cell becomes active, it reproduces the viral RNA which encodes viral proteins, and millions of new complete virus particles (virions) are formed to infect other susceptible hosts. It is this retrovirus which is indicative of the acquired immunodeficiency syndrome since "HIV or antibodies to it are found in essentially all patients with AIDS."[29]

HIV transmission occurs when infected cells enter the bloodstream. Once in the bloodstream, they can be found in various bodily solutions including, but not limited to, blood, semen, and vaginal secretions. Primary cells targeted for infection appear to be T4 lymphocytes, monocyte-macrophage cells, certain brain and spinal cord cell populations, and colorectal epithelial cells. T4 lymphocytes and monocyte-macrophage cells are essential to the proper functioning of the human immune system. It is believed that colorectal cell infection may play an important role in homosexual transmission of the virus, while the effect of HIV on brain and spinal cord cell populations is less certain. After invading the body, HIV–even while appearing to lie dormant–may sufficiently impair or disrupt normal cell processes to allow for progression to the various stages of HIV infection, or to the development of full-blown AIDS.[30] It is now believed that rather than lying dormant after transmission, HIV begins replicating in the lymph system.[31]

Psychosocial

In addition to infecting the brain and central nervous system, HIV may produce psychological manifestations which are secondary to medical diagnosis. Many psychiatric presentations in HIV-infected individuals result from the stresses related to the knowledge of infection.[32] These may be divided into adjustment reactions and disorders, affective disorders, and schizophreniform and paranoid disorders. Adjustment reactions involve expressions of anger, anxiety, depression, despair, grief, and guilt. These emotions tend to be less severe in nature and do not impair normal functioning. When these features endure and become excessive or intense, they are termed adjustment disorders. Major depressive disorders are the primary manifestation of an abnormal affective state and are more prevalent in individuals at advanced stages of progression through the CDC categories of HIV infection. An increased risk of suicide very often accompanies affective disorders. Although not easily discernible, nonorganic psychoses–schizophreniform, paranoid psychoses, depressive psychoses, and hypomania–have been detected in some patients, but tend to be limited to later stages of the illness.

In view of the legal, medical, and psychological complexities of the AIDS epidemic, coping mechanisms and sources of comfort are an obvious necessity. "Traditionally, in times of illness, religious communities have been an effective support system for individuals, their families, and friends."[33] However, this is not always the case with HIV infection and AIDS. This divergence from religion's traditional role in the provision of support in times of crisis is due predominantly to the modes of HIV transmission and the nature of groups perceived to be at high risk for infection. Blame–rather than support–has been laid upon gay men throughout the pandemic. This may be evinced in the decrees put forth by various religious leaders. For example, the Anglican Dean of Sydney, Australia, was quoted as saying "Gays have blood on their hands"; the former president of the American Southern Baptist Convention, Charles Stanley, proclaimed, "AIDS is God indicating his displeasure toward a sinful lifestyle"; and Jerry Falwell claimed, "AIDS is the wrath of God upon homosexuals," while yet another religious publication "predicts that God will not permit science to find a cure for AIDS because homosexuality shall not be accepted nor condoned by the Eternal Father even if he has to send another plague upon you."[34] Cardinal John J. O'Connor, Archbishop of New York, decreed in his keynote address at an AIDS conference organized by the Pontifical Council for Health Care Workers in Rome that "The greatest danger done to persons with AIDS is done by the dishonesty of those health-care professionals who refuse to confront the moral dimensions of sexual aberrations or drug abuse."[35] Despite the arguments which can, and have been made against the idea that AIDS is a punishment from God–why has God singled out homosexuals as those deserving AIDS rather than other groups of sinners, why is the United States the only country where the majority of AIDS cases involve homosexual men, why has God waited until now to punish homosexuals as same-sex relationships can be traced back to ancient times, why are male homosexuals more deserving of this disease than lesbians–there are still those who continue to hold this belief.[36] It is understandable how this negative concept contributes to the stigmatization associated with HIV and AIDS.

Conversely, there are some religious leaders–such as Mother Teresa–who have embraced the teachings of the New Testament of the Bible which promote charity, compassion, pity, and self-sacrifice. These teachings do not include a disclaimer based on a sick individual's mode of infection or the nature of his or her lifestyle. Personal spirituality, as well as religious denomination, may continue to provide solace to HIV-infected individuals in instances where community leaders have the forethought to overcome unwarranted fears and established prejudices. This may be witnessed in such works as the statement from the November 1989 U.S. Catholic Bishops' Meeting, "Called to Compassion and Responsibility: A Response to the HIV/AIDS Crisis."[37]

Just as personal spirituality and religious denomination contribute to the complexities of the epidemic, so does society at large. Perhaps one of the greatest societal contributions to the stigmatization associated with AIDS–given that the gay community continues to be the most affected in the United States–is the manifestation of deep-seated fear, misunderstanding, and prejudice as homophobia. AIDS, for better or worse, has increased the visibility of the homosexual community. This increased visibility has not necessarily yielded greater acceptance–tolerance should be differentiated from acceptance–as may be evinced in the recent increase in hate crimes directed toward homosexuals. Further, "the negative attitudes toward homosexual men and women that pervade American society often lead to rejection and alienation that affects the gay person's self-esteem."[38] Rejection, alienation, isolation, and damaged self-esteem may, and often do, play key roles in contributing to the decisions a person makes (consciously or unconsciously) regarding treatment, and even the ultimate success of that treatment. Attitudes similar to homophobia exist for other groups–such as IV drug users and prostitutes–perceived to be at risk for HIV infection. It is important to remember that "the psychosocial impact of AIDS on the lives of persons with the disease or at risk for it includes the magnification of the preexisting socially condoned antipathy toward them."[39]

PREVENTION AND CONTROL

As there is currently neither a known cure for AIDS nor a vaccine to prevent HIV infection, education is the primary means available to combat the onslaught of the epidemic. The major thrust of the various educational programs has been to promote health for the general public. These educational promotions have included health education messages, safe sex campaigns, and accurate information concerning the dangers of drug abuse. A major key to the success of any of these projects is the availability of timely, relevant, valid information produced in an appealing manner and in a language comprehensible to the target audience. This has resulted in AIDS education television commercials, radio spots, advertisements on public transportation systems, and presentations to institutions and organizations. However, these educational campaigns–produced and presented in an effort to control the spread of the epidemic–have met with considerable resistance and have been fraught with controversy.

AIDS education is an elective process. Although information is available, people cannot be forced to learn the facts surrounding HIV and AIDS. Laws do not exist to coerce individuals to become knowledgeable about modes of HIV transmission. Quite the contrary, many government-funded programs have restricted the use of explicit information or demonstrations. How does one explain safe sex without discussing sex? What does it mean to use protection? Although there has been considerable discussion regarding the creation and implementation of statutes and legislation to control HIV-infected individuals (through mandatory testing or quarantine, for example), there is limited evidence to show that policies reflect a more aggressive stance on ascertaining the facts regarding infection, modes of transmission, or progression from HIV infection to AIDS.

Contact tracing–which violates the patient/physician trust–poses a significant problem for the medical profession. This trust, in addition to being one of the cornerstones of medical ethics, is one of the allures of voluntary HIV antibody testing. The knowledge that this confidence is going to be breached has the potential to negate any positive attitudes about testing by choice.

As previously stated, AIDS education is an elective process. Even though data are available to help prevent infection, many individuals who are aware of the facts concerning AIDS and HIV choose not to apply this information to their own lives. Considering the spectrum of those infected, the prevalence of an attitude that AIDS is a gay, white, male disease is astounding. (White males exposed through homosexual/bisexual contact currently account for approximately 45 percent of the total reported cases of AIDS in the United States.[40]) Similarly, the belief that certain groups or people are immune–the invincibility of youth–continues to hold sway. In fact, the vast majority of those individuals developing AIDS in their twenties were probably infected during their teens, since the median incubation period in adults is seven to ten years. Certain populations have adopted a defeatist attitude toward contagion. This may be attributable to the notion that the pleasure sought far outweighs the risk taken. The lack of concern or failure of educational efforts is painfully obvious with each new diagnosis.

Many of the issues associated with HIV and AIDS–drug abuse, sexuality, prostitution, homosexuality–touch on sensitive religious areas. Many religious leaders feel that discussing these sensitive issues is tantamount to condoning them. The argument that AIDS is a punishment from God has bound more than one set of hands in the religious community where education is concerned. The difficulties in providing accurate and complete AIDS education without encroaching on religious beliefs is obvious. The source of much of the difficulty rests in the judgmental view most organized religions currently hold concerning prevalent modes of transmission.

Social barriers are perhaps the greatest obstacles in the path of effective AIDS education. Since the acquired immunodeficiency syndrome involves individuals who may not be considered participants in mainstream society (gays, IV drug users, and prostitutes) and because AIDS concerns issues which put people very much ill-at-ease (death, sexuality, drug abuse, and homosexuality), it is not surprising that whole sectors of society censor AIDS educational efforts. For example, North American society is typically considered to be both death-denying and sex-denying; and yet AIDS has brought both of these issues to the forefront of daily existence. The reluctance to discuss these important, yet closeted, issues pervades society, even to the point of sheltering children–who may very well be at risk for infection–from being exposed to the truth concerning HIV and AIDS.

DEATH AND AIDS

Many people find it hard to face and accept death–both in others and in themselves. However, this lack of acceptance seems to be even more exaggerated, perhaps because of the nature of the death and those involved, with the acquired immunodeficiency syndrome. The onset of the disease or infection which ultimately causes an AIDS-related death may be acute or chronic, just as the death itself may occur quickly or be prolonged. Some of the diseases or manifestations of the human immunodeficiency virus–Kaposi's sarcoma with its purplish lesions, cytomegalovirus retinitis (CMV retinitis) which may ultimately cause blindness, or HIV wasting syndrome which may result in emaciation–may be severely disfiguring. Other diseases–such as HIV encephalopathy or toxoplasmosis–affect the brain and central nervous system, which may render the individual devoid of mental capacities.

These excruciating deaths–often intensely painful and almost always terribly distressing–are viewed with trepidation because of the nature of the people afflicted. More often than not, AIDS strikes individuals in the prime of their lives. It is difficult enough to cope with death when the person is elderly; but when death involves people who have substantial parts of their lives before them, it is almost beyond comprehension. All too often within the AIDS epidemic, parents are burying their children rather than children burying their parents. Moreover, people in the prime of their lives are suffering the loss of friends and lovers as AIDS continues to claim more and more lives.

With such a high case-fatality rate, issues concerning the dying process–for those directly involved as well as their survivors–cannot help but be of significant concern within the AIDS arena. Dying an AIDS-related death is complicated by the various legal, medical, psychological, religious, and social issues associated with the disease. Moreover, in the case of this illness, death does not constitute the end of the disease. AIDS has managed to transgress life and the limitations of the human body.

CONCLUSION

The AIDS pandemic is riddled with various issues–medical, legal, social, religious, psychological–that complicate its very nature. The constellation of diseases and opportunistic infections associated with HIV and AIDS have created a myriad of obstacles to medical care, and have exacerbated clinical decision making concerning the treatment of infected patients. In addition to the complex biomedical nature of the human immunodeficiency virus and the acquired immunodeficiency syndrome, this epidemic has fostered legal debate and forced into existence decisions concerning HIV/AIDS that set disease-specific legal precedents. This disease-specific litigation is predominantly a result of the social perception of the epidemic and those individuals who have been affected by the illness. Society tends not to be empathetic or sympathetic toward HIV-infected individuals. The virus, due in part to modes of transmission, remains a societal taboo, as do members of most categories considered initially to be high risk–homosexuals, drug abusers, and employees of the sex industry. Similarly, most formal religions do not condone the actions that facilitate viral transmission of the disease. Some religious leaders continue to advocate that AIDS is a just punishment from God for immoral actions. These medical, legal, social, and religious issues contribute significantly to psychological unrest among HIV-infected individuals, as do the neurological disorders associated with the disease and the prospect of impending death as the illness progresses.

Just as the AIDS epidemic is complicated by the medical,

legal, social, religious, and psychological factors associated with the disease, AIDS-related information is intrinsically entwined with the substance of those factors and constrained by their structure. This body of information is circumscribed by the various complexities that directly affect HIV-infected individuals, resulting in data that may not exist or may not be accessible. Therefore, it is necessary to consult various sources of information, including those that are not HIV/AIDS-specific, and apply that information based on the construct of the epidemic.

REFERENCES

1. Foucault M. *The Birth of the Clinic: An Archaeology of Medical Perception,* trans. AM Sheridan Smith. New York: Vintage Books, 1975. 3-20.

2. Ibid.: 126.

3. Ibid.: 16.

4. Ibid.: 20.

5. Selik RM, Buehler JW, Karon JM, Chamberland ME, Berkelman RL. Impact of the 1987 revision of the case definition of acquired immune deficiency syndrome in the United States. *Journal of Acquired Immune Deficiency Syndromes*. 3(1):73-82, 1990.

6. CDC. Revision of the CDC surveillance case definition for acquired immunodeficiency syndrome. Council of State and Territorial Epidemiologists; AIDS Program, Center for Infectious Diseases. *MMWR–Morbidity & Mortality Weekly Report*. 36(Suppl 1):1S-15S, 1987 Aug 14.

7. Soskolne CL. Proportion of new AIDS case reports attributable to the 1987 CDC revised surveillance case definition: Canada-United States differences. *Canadian Journal of Public Health*. 80:380-381, 1989 Sep/Oct.

8. Payne SF, Rutherford GW, Lemp GF, Clevenger AC. Effect of the revised AIDS case definition on AIDS reporting in San Francisco: Evidence of increased reporting in intravenous drug users. *AIDS*. 4(4):335-339, 1990 Apr.

9. Centers for Disease Control and Prevention. 1993 Revised Classification System for HIV Infection and Expanded Surveillance Case Definition for AIDS Among Adolescents and Adults. *MMWR*. 41(RR-17):1-19, 1992.

10. Caussy D, Goedert JJ. The epidemiology of human immunodeficiency virus and acquired immunodeficiency syndrome. *Seminars in Oncology*. 17:244-250, 1990 Jun.

11. Centers for Disease Control and Prevention. *HIV/AIDS Surveillance Report*. 5(4):1-33, 1994.

12. Ibid.

13. Caussy D, Goedert JJ. The epidmiology of human immundeficiency virus and acquired immunodeficiency syndrome. *Seminars in Oncology.* 17:244-250, 1990 Jun.

14. Centers for Disease Control and Prevention. *HIV/AIDS Surveillance Report.* 5(4):1-33, 1994.

15. Ibid.

16. Caussy D, Goedert JJ. The epidemiology of human immunodeficiency virus and acquired immunodeficiency syndrome. *Seminars in Oncology.* 17:244-250, 1990 Jun.

17. Ibid.

18. Centers for Disease Control and Prevention. *HIV/AIDS Surveillance Report.* 5(4):1-33, 1994.

19. Caussy D, Goedert JJ. The epidemiology of human immunodeficiency virus and acquired immunodeficiency syndrome. *Seminars in Oncology.* 17:244-250, 1990 Jun.

20. Volberding PA. Recent advances in the medical management of early HIV disease. *Journal of General Internal Medicine.* 6:S7-S11, 1991 Jan/Feb.

21. Cates W. Acquired immunodeficiency syndrome, sexually transmitted diseases, and epidemiology. *American Journal of Epidemiology.* 131:749-758, 1990 May.

22. CDC. Classification system for human T-lymphotropic virus type III/ lymphadenophthy-associated virus infections. *MMWR–Morbidity & Mortality Weekly Report.* 35(20):334-339, 1986 May 23.

23. Redfield RR, Wright DC, Tramont ED. The Walter Reed staging classification for HTLV-III/LAV infection. *New England Journal of Medicine.* 314(2):131-132, 1986 Jan 9.

24. Centers for Disease Control and Prevention. 1993 revised classification system for HIV infection and expanded surveillance case definition for AIDS among adolescents and adults. *MMWR.* 41(RR-17):1-19, 1992.

25. Gostin, LO. The AIDS litigation project: A national review of court and human rights decisions, Part I: The social impact of AIDS. *JAMA.* 263(14):1961-1970, 1990 Apr 11.

26. Bayer R, Gostin L. Legal and ethical issues relating to AIDS. *Bulletin of the Pan American Health Organization.* 24(4):454-468, 1990.

27. Markowitz JC, Perry SW. Medical overview of HIV infection, in *Psychiatric Aspects of AIDS and HIV Infection*, SM Goldfinger (ed.). San Francisco: Jossey-Bass, 1990.

28. CDC. *HIV/AIDS Surveillance Report.* 6(1):1-27, 1994.

29. Markowitz JC, Perry SW. Medical overview of HIV infection, in *Psychiatric Aspects of AIDS and HIV Infection*, SM Goldfinger (ed.). San Francisco: Jossey-Bass, 1990.

30. Groopman JE. The acquired immunodeficiency syndrome, in *Cecil Textbook of Medicine*, JB Wyngaarden and LH Smith (ed.). 18th ed. Philadelphia: W.B. Saunders, 1988.

31. Feinberg, MB. HIV disease: New tools, new understanding. *BETA: Bulletin of Experimental Treatment for AIDS*. 41-43, 1994 Sep.

32. Miller D, Riccio M. Non-organic psychiatric and psychosocial syndromes associated with HIV-1 infection and disease. *AIDS*. 4(5):381-388, 1990 May.

33. Shelp EE, DuBose ER, Sunderland, RH. The infrastructure of religious communities: A neglected resource for care for people with AIDS. *American Journal of Public Health*. 80:970-972, 1990.

34. Ross JW. Ethics and the language of AIDS, in *AIDS Ethics and Public Policy*, C Pierce and D Vandeveer (ed.) . Belmont, CA: Wadsworth, 1988.

35. O'Connor JJ. Who will care for the AIDS victims? *Origins*. 19:544-548, 1990 Jan 18.

36. Murphy TF. Is AIDS a just punishment? *Journal of Medical Ethics*. 14:154-160, 1988.

37. U.S. Catholic Bishops. Called to compassion and responsibility: A response to the HIV/AIDS crisis. *Origins*. 19:421, 423-436, 1989 Nov 30.

38. Govoni LA. Psychosocial issues of AIDS in the nursing care of homosexual men and their significant others. *Nursing Clinics of North America*. 23:749-765, 1988 Dec.

39. Friedlander AH, Arthur RJ. A diagnosis of AIDS: Understanding the psychosocial impact. *Oral Surgery, Oral Medicine, Oral Pathology*. 65(6):680-684, 1988 Jun.

40. CDC. *HIV/AIDS Surveillance Report*. 6(1):1-27, 1994.

Chapter 2

HIV/AIDS Information

THE INFORMATION OF DISEASE OR THE DISEASE OF INFORMATION: AN INTEGRAL RELATIONSHIP

The body of information concerning a disease exists to describe the illness, classify the malady, and discuss the affected individuals. This pool of knowledge brings life to the disease; for without information–data consisting of signs and symbols used to describe the illness–the pathological remains invisible. A reciprocal relationship exists, however, since there would be no information if there were no disease. Moreover, the information concerning a disease is bound by the life of that pathological condition. The stigma associated with a particular illness directly affects the body of information produced to describe that malady. Information is circumscribed by the same constraints that bind the disease itself.

INFORMATION AND DISEASE

If one examines the paradigm of information-knowledge-wisdom, information forms the first step in the attainment of knowledge. Information is what is used to affect a decision; while knowledge connotes understanding, it is with the implication that not all information is understood. Knowledge represents a higher degree of certainty or validity than information, whereas wisdom implies insight. Education follows this same paradigm, as it is information that forms the basis for all enlightenment. If information is needed anywhere, it is needed in the fight against the human immunodeficiency virus and the acquired immunodeficiency syndrome. People must be informed in order to understand the reality and the gravity of the AIDS pandemic. The importance of providing timely, correct information in the AIDS arena can not be overemphasized. Education is currently the only weapon available to stem the spread of the epidemic and to foster support to those already affected.

The AIDS pandemic is unlike any other phenomena witnessed by modern society. It has been termed the greatest public health concern of our era and has been compared to such illnesses as cancer, polio, syphilis, and the plague. However, most known diseases or infections pale in comparison to the severity and complexity of this modern public health dilemma. It is currently estimated that millions of people worldwide are infected with the human immunodeficiency virus, the virus believed to cause the acquired immunodeficiency syndrome. Moreover, the record of documented cases of AIDS continues to expand as do the number of AIDS-related deaths. Statistics concerning HIV and AIDS, however, are understated at best, given the medical complexities of the disease coupled with the legal, moral, psychological, religious, and social implications of an AIDS diagnosis.

One of the things that continues to differentiate the AIDS epidemic from other diseases is the complex nature of the information associated with AIDS and HIV. This is further exacerbated by the nontraditional modes of information creation and consumption within the AIDS arena, and by the diverse backgrounds of consumers of AIDS-related data. In working with this body of information, it is imperative to be cognizant of the peculiarities in the paradigm of creator-seeker-provider as they differ from the traditional model. In addition, the amount of information concerning the pandemic is expanding proportionately to the number of reported AIDS cases. However, much of this data continues to be published and distributed outside of traditional publishing channels. For this reason, access to existing information can be difficult. Moreover, the comprehensiveness and quality of available AIDS-related information continues to function as a point of contention among individuals working in this area. To further exacerbate the situation, the pandemic has spawned its own vernacular–one comprised of scientific terminology and vocabularies reflective of the populations most affected.

RELATIONSHIP OF INFORMATION CREATOR AND CONSUMER

When working with AIDS-related information, it is necessary to consider the relationship between the information creator and the information consumer. "Traditionally, it has been the responsibility of the researcher to describe phenomena and disseminate information, while the policymaker and the practitioner are charged with applying this knowledge. The AIDS crisis challenges this traditional division and forges stronger and more effective working partnerships."[1] Consumers of data concerning HIV and AIDS are very often producers of this same information. Through efforts such as the Community Research Initiative, individuals who are HIV infected or at risk for infection may be directly involved in biomedical research and the publication of research findings. The health care consumer becomes an active participant in the research process. Similarly, it is necessary to consider the popular consumer as well as the health care professional when approaching this body of information, since a significant portion of AIDS information consumers are highly educated and well-informed. The extent of the knowledge base possessed by an individual affected by the epidemic has direct impact on the interaction between health care professional and health care consumer. It is not uncommon for a person with HIV to be aware of treatment advances prior to his or her health care provider, or to be involved in information networks so as to remain informed where issues regarding this illness are concerned. These informed consumers, together with structured AIDS organizations, have proven to be formidable opponents to existing policies and practices in the health care and information industries. They have challenged community misperceptions, business and societal standards, local service providers, government agencies, and officials in an effort to serve the needs of those individuals affected by the epidemic and to combat the spread of the disease. For example, this influence may be seen in its impact on the peer review and publication process–most major medical journals now have given priority status to the expeditious publication of AIDS-related studies–and its legitimatization of the alternative press.

Conversely, many individuals belonging to high-risk populations–adolescents, IV drug users, minorities–may not be well-educated about the pandemic or may lack the ability to read at a level sufficient to educate themselves. Approximately 50 percent of health care consumers have difficulty reading, or are unable to read, educational instructions written at a fifth grade level;[2] and at least 20 percent of consumers are unable to read instructional materials at all.[3] Studies indicate that ethnic minorities from impoverished backgrounds, particularly blacks and Hispanics, are more likely to have difficulty reading.[4] The correlation between education and disease prevention can be illustrated in the context of the human immunodeficiency virus and the acquired immunodeficiency syndrome by examining the number of reported cases of AIDS among the African-American community in the United States. While blacks constitute approximately 12 percent of the U.S. population, they account for more than 30 percent of AIDS cases.[5] And Hispanics account for more than 17 percent of U.S. AIDS cases. Moreover, it has been found that

"Blacks and Hispanics have the least knowledge about AIDS and are more likely than other ethnic groups to participate in high-risk sexual practices."[6]

Complicating this situation more, the pandemic has created its own body of professionals; and many AIDS professionals–those individuals working directly with populations affected by the epidemic–possess neither a biomedical nor an information background. Initially, most AIDS service organizations and community-based organizations were founded by individuals affected by the disease and those perceived to be at risk for infection. The main criteria for service was a willingness and desire to help, not the nature of educational and professional experience. These organizations, which frequently continue to be staffed by individuals from diverse backgrounds, have grown into powerful entities that provide invaluable contributions to the community through the support services they offer. However, the lack of a biomedical or information background has had an impact on this body of professionals and the services they provide. Some of the duplication of AIDS-related materials may be attributable to a knowledge deficit concerning existing materials. If the availability of information resources is not apparent, the assumption is often made that such materials do not exist, and that it is necessary to create them. In addition, this may account for some instances of not disseminating the most up-to-date information or not utilizing the most appropriate information technologies. Thus, the relationship between information creator, seeker, and provider is of considerable importance within this realm of health care.

AIDS-RELATED INFORMATION

Initially, AIDS-related information was limited in size, scope, and availability.[7] Research itself was limited in the early years of the epidemic, and many publications concerning the results of the research that was being conducted were often tied up in the peer review and publication process. In order to fill this void, individuals affected by the epidemic began to alter the traditional model of publication and distribution by producing information at the local level. A great deal of AIDS-related information has been—and continues to be—produced by, and distributed through, the popular press and/or community-based organizations. Examples of information produced at the local level include directories, training manuals, issue-specific guidelines for working with HIV-infected individuals, current drug and therapeutic information, educational materials, pamphlets, and brochures, as well as compilations of technical data gleaned from traditional biomedical resources and translated into layperson's terms. This wealth of information, though, is often overlooked since it is not part of standard clinical information resources. While this body of information may not constitute the typical source from which to pool relevant data, it does serve a valid function within the AIDS arena. For example, AIDS newsletters, having evolved from an underground press network to a recognized information resource, supply data to individuals directly affected by HIV and AIDS, as well as to the health care establishment working in this area, that cannot be found in official biomedical publications.[8] Some examples of these newsletters include Project Inform's *P.I. Perspective; Treatment Issues* produced by the Gay Men's Health Crisis; and the San Francisco AIDS Foundation's *BETA (Bulletin of Experimental Treatments for AIDS)*.

Currently, there is an abundance of information concerning HIV and AIDS. Information is produced at the local, national, and international level, and is published in both the popular and scientific press. As the incidence rate of HIV infection and subsequent development of AIDS continues to rise, the amount of AIDS-related information steadily increases. It has been observed that the number of documented cases of AIDS doubles every ten or 11 months, with the body of literature concerning the epidemic doubling in volume every 22 months.[9] Sources and resources of information concerning the pandemic currently run the gamut of those available for data dissemination, including print, audio-visual, and electronic formats. In addition to AIDS-related books, journals, videos, databases, electronic bulletin boards, and messaging systems, there are photodocumentaries, poems, plays, films, and archival memorabilia including a quilt honoring those who have died from AIDS-related causes. There are various directories, such as *AIDS Information Sourcebook,*[10] *How to Find Information About AIDS,*[11] or *Learning AIDS,*[12] designed specifically to assist information seekers in accessing data.

The proliferation of information concerning the human immunodeficiency virus and the acquired immunodeficiency syndrome, nevertheless, is often neither easily accessible nor readily comprehensive. Since AIDS-related information is produced in almost every format and is both produced and distributed by various individuals and organizations, access can easily become difficult. The very nature of the epidemic–one that impinges on many disciplines–further complicates the organization of the information. AIDS literature is scattered, and important papers are published in a wide range of primary journals. One study found that out of 628 journals known to have published AIDS literature, 50 percent of AIDS-related articles were concentrated in 35 journals and the remaining 50 percent scattered within 593 journals.[13] This scattering and seepage has direct implications concerning dissemination and retrieval of relevant data. It may be necessary to consult multiple sources of information rather than limiting perusal to a selective few. The concept of "core" versus "fringe" journals may not be valid where HIV/AIDS is concerned, given the breadth of the literature coupled with the scatter of data. Moreover, the notion of a single authoritative resource–or even several authoritative resources–may be questioned as a result of the scattering and seepage of data. Similarly, many online databases can be used to retrieve information, but the user must be aware of the strengths and weaknesses of each and their varying emphases.[14] The results of a bibliometric study concerning the scientific literature of AIDS specific to women indicated that the journal scatter for this subset of literature differs from that of the general literature, and that the information indexed in six key databases demonstrated little overlap.[15] It is necessary to understand database content relative to the nature of the information query so as to know when it is more appropriate to search an AIDS-specific database as opposed to a general biomedical, legal, or psychosocial database. With regard to specialized electronic HIV/AIDS-specific resources, it becomes critical to develop further understanding of subject matter in order to determine which is the more suitable source of information (e.g., the AIDS Database produced by the Bureau of Hygiene and Tropical Diseases as opposed to the National Library of Medicine's AIDSLINE; AIDSDRUGS versus AIDSTRIALS; or *The AIDS Knowledge Base* rather than many of the other HIV/AIDS-specific databases). A further impediment to access is the lack of standardization in cataloging and indexing practices for AIDS-related information. Much of the information produced by AIDS service organizations and community-based organizations is neither cataloged nor indexed. Thus, the information remains invisible to those unaware of its existence. Moreover, in spite of the multitude of information currently available concerning AIDS and HIV, access often remains restricted because the epidemic has publicly re-presented and exposed many subjects (death, drug abuse, bisexuality, homosexuality, or human sexuality) which the general populace has historically chosen to either censor or ignore.[16] In addition, the epidemic is in constant flux, making it neither uncommon for information to be outdated nor for information to be withheld from the public for a period of time. The medical complexities of this intricate disease–further exacerbated by the legal, ethical, psychological, religious, and social issues that surround it–impact the body of information concerning it. Although an abundance of information exists, the way in which an individual seeks out that information may color his or her perception of the pandemic. The subject matter itself may directly affect access to that information, making availability less than apparent. In those instances when the information exists but is not available or accessible, one is faced more with a knowledge deficit rather than an information deficit.

Even with the expansive amount of AIDS-related information currently available, there are still many omissions. In one study, it was found that "examples of major information breaches included: asymptomatic seropositives' psychological and clinical management; updates on clinical trials; perinatal and pediatric issues; general gynecological care of the HIV-positive female; HIV-related nursing care and research; methodologies for working with Hispanic and other minority clients; undocumented women from Mexico and Central America; reaching individuals at high risk in low incidence areas; correctional facilities and HIV/AIDS–particularly adolescent-oriented facilities; the use of epidemiology to devise and direct programs; intervening in the family; ethical concerns; death, dying, and grief; involvement of the clergy; and ways to improve cooperation among CBO's."[17] While some of these information deficits have begun to be addressed, many gaps continue to exist. Since significant gaps do exist in the currently available AIDS-specific information, it is always important to research the topic outside of the AIDS arena and then apply that information to HIV and AIDS based on the constructs of the epidemic.

As well as not being comprehensive, existing AIDS-related information has been questioned concerning its quality. Often educational materials are written with little regard for the target audience and with insufficient preparation and research by the author and/or compiler. A prime example of this phenomenon–disregarding the consumer for whom the information is prepared–is documented in the results of a study that found most instructions for condom use "required at least reading at the level of a high school graduate and none required less than a tenth grade level."[18] This would tend to ignore the fact that many adolescents have engaged in sexual activity prior to this age, and that functionally illiterate people engage in sex at all. Another study asserted that:

> Reading levels of materials are too high for many target audiences; that a lack of material exists for IV drug users, church communities, gay and bisexual minorities, women of color, and HIV-positive asymptomatic persons; that translations and the cultural sensitivity of materials are inadequate; that the body of primary material is repetitive; that there is a lack of interactive material–over 50% of the material reviewed utilized formats (brochures, PSA's, posters) which were not conducive to an in-depth presentation of information encouraging participant interaction.[19]

The medical, legal, psychological, social, religious, financial, and human complexities associated with AIDS have tended to add to the mystique and fear surrounding the epidemic. Since work is being done at various levels to unravel these complications (in order to clarify public understanding of the disease, discover a vaccine to prevent HIV infection, and ultimately find a cure for AIDS) information is often outdated upon publication. Outdated information is of course potentially dangerous in the fight against the spread of the epidemic, unless the recipient is aware that the data may no longer be current, comprehensive, or even correct. "Because so many public attitudes and private actions are conditioned by medical and scientific information about AIDS, that information must be presented accurately, comprehensively and in perspective about how AIDS is and is not spread."[20] Therapeutic issues, in addition to prevention and control, are closely tied to the accuracy of HIV and AIDS-related data. The currency and comprehensiveness of this information directly impacts on the lives of those individuals at risk for infection and those individuals currently affected by this disease.

When examining AIDS-related information as it relates to the general public's understanding of AIDS, it is important to realize that "most people rely on television, newspapers, and magazines for general information on AIDS, followed by radio, brochures, fliers, pamphlets, and word of mouth. Only when their information needs become more pressing do Americans turn to physicians, health professionals, or AIDS professionals for specific information on the detection, treatment, and research on AIDS."[21] Thus, the manner in which an individual seeks information concerning the disease may affect his or her perception of the facts surrounding HIV and AIDS. It has been found that:

> There are significant differences based on information sources. Television viewers tend to perceive lower risk, are less likely to want HIV-infected people on the job, and are more apt to believe that medical authorities know less and are telling less than do those whose primary information source is either print or authoritative. Education has had little impact on this population concerning attitudes toward HIV-infected workers or on risk perception.[22]

In spite of the complex nature of AIDS-related data, coupled with the intricate relationship between information creator and consumer, much of the body of information concerning HIV and AIDS continues to be produced in medical or specialized verbiage (including jargon adopted from high-risk populations) that is not readily comprehensible to the information seeker. As well as including terminology that may not be understood, the vocabulary employed often assumes an altered meaning when applied to HIV and AIDS. Because this vocabulary–consisting of a combination of both technical and common terms–is utilized by such a diverse group of individuals with varying degrees of education and experience, difficulties may arise for the layperson in understanding medical, pharmaceutical, and technical terminology and for health care professionals with population-specific jargon adopted by individuals working with or affected by the epidemic. Moreover, often there is a general lack of consistency in the use of terminology that makes navigation in the sea of HIV/AIDS information even more difficult. Although the acronym AIDS originally stood for acquired immune deficiency syndrome, it evolved into the now commonly accepted form acquired immunodeficiency syndrome. Nonetheless, the initial form–acquired immune deficiency syndrome–continues to be used, as does the acronym, in addition to the commonly accepted articulation. Similarly, AIDS and HIV–along with various counterparts–are often used interchangeably in spite of various differences. In essence, the pandemic has spawned its own vernacular–with little consistency or precision among users–and this vernacular further muddies the waters of the AIDS information continuum.

CONCLUSION

Although a proliferation of AIDS-related information currently exists, access to that information continues to be riddled with complexities not unlike those associated with the disease itself. The communications gap within the AIDS arena constitutes a significant contribution to the difficulties associated with accessing available data. For the health care professional, the complex nature of the information may contribute to a lack of understanding of those individuals directly affected by the epidemic, a lack of awareness of services currently available to those people suffering with the disease, or a lack of knowledge regarding therapeutic advances. For the general public or the AIDS professional without a biomedical or information background, these complexities may contribute to a lack of awareness and understanding of available therapies, or even foster the continued increase in the incidence rate of HIV and AIDS. In light of the intricacies of AIDS-related information, and given the diverse nature of consumers of that information, it is expected that the AIDS pandemic will continue to foster a nontraditional model of information creation and dissemination. For at a time when information is the only weapon available to stem the spread of the epidemic and to promote potential support and treatment to those already affected, access to, and understanding of, existing data remain crucial, as does the continued need to strengthen the body of information (both in content and organization) associated with this chronic illness.

REFERENCES

1. Michal-Johnson P, Bowen SP. AIDS and communication: A matter of influence. *AIDS & Public Policy Journal.* 4(1):1-2, 1989.

2. Doak C, Doak L. Patient comprehension profiles: Recent findings and strategies. *Patient Counseling and Health Education.* 3:101-106, 1980.

3. Mohammed M. Patients' understanding of written health instructions. *Nursing Research.* 13:232-235, 1964.

4. Ledbetter C, Johnson D. AIDS: Reading level analysis of understanding AIDS. *AIDS & Public Policy Journal.* 4(3):168-170, 1989.

5. Centers for Disease Control and Prevention. *HIV/AIDS Surveillance Report.* 6(1):1-27, 1994.

6. Ledbetter C, Johnson D. AIDS: Reading level analysis of understanding AIDS. *AIDS & Public Policy Journal.* 4(3):168-170, 1989.

7. SantaVicca EF. Acquired immune deficiency syndrome (AIDS): An annotated bibliography for librarians. *Reference Services Review.* 15:45-67, 1987.

8. Bishop K. Underground press leads way on AIDS advice. *The New York Times.* 1991 Dec 16.

9. Sengupta IN, Kumari L. Bibliometric analysis of AIDS literature. *Scientometrics.* 20:297-315, 1991.

10. Malinowski HR and Perry GJ (eds.). *The AIDS Information Sourcebook, 1993-94,* 4th ed. Phoenix, AZ: Oryx Press, 1993.

11. Huber JT (ed.). *How to Find Information About AIDS.* 2nd ed. New York: The Haworth Press, 1992.

12. Halleron T, Pisaneschi J, and Trapani M (eds.). *Learning AIDS: An Information Resource Directory.* 2nd ed. New York: American Foundation for AIDS Research, 1989.

13. Sengupta IN, Kumari L. Bibliometric analysis of AIDS literature. *Scientometrics.* 20:297-315, 1991.

14. Roberts S, Shepherd L, Wade J. The scientific and clinical literature of AIDS: Development, bibliographic control and retrieval. *Health Libraries Review.* 4:197-218, 1987.

15. Gillaspy ML, Huber JT. A look at the scientific literature specific to women: A vital link in health information for the global village. *Medical Library Association 95th Annual Meeting. 37,* 1995 May 7-10.

16. SantaVicca EF. AIDS in the minds of librarians: Opinion, perception, and misperception. *Library Journal.* 112:113-115, 1987.

17. Ouren J, Pittman-Lindeman M. Information gaps among HIV service providers. *International Conference on AIDS VI. 465,* 1990 Jun 20-23.

18. Richwald GA, Wamsley MA, Coulson, AH, Morisky DE. Are condom instructions readable? Results of a readability study. *Public Health Reports.* 103(4):355-359, 1988.

19. Halleron-Tweedley T, Ranieri A. Qualitative and quantitative analysis of AIDS education materials. *International Conference on AIDS IV.* 297, 1990 Jun 20-23.

20. Lunin LF. AIDS and information: in time of plague. *Bulletin of the American Society of Information Science.* 14:15-16, 1988.

21. Kirby DG, Harvell TA. U.S. government information policy and the AIDS epidemic. *Government Publications Review.* 16:157-171, 1989.

22. Sumser J, Gerbert B, Maguire B. The American public's sources of information about AIDS. *International Conference on AIDS IV.* 299, 1990 Jun 20-23.

Chapter 3

HIV/AIDS Information Resources and Services

BREADTH AND DEPTH

While data concerning the human immunodeficiency virus and the acquired immunodeficiency syndrome may not be readily accessible in all instances, specialized information resources do exist. Many libraries and information centers have recognized the need for HIV/AIDS-specific services and have sought to fulfill client needs based on the mission of the individual library or organization. Services vary in nature, from the creation and maintenance of bibliographies concerning various aspects of the epidemic, to the provision of computer programs that facilitate determining whether or not to be tested for antibodies to the human immunodeficiency virus, based on risk for infection. Special information centers such as the National AIDS Hotline or the National AIDS Clearinghouse provide reference services and/or educational materials at no charge. There are also a variety of AIDS-specific electronic sources of information ranging in nature from online databases such as AIDSLINE, AIDSTRIALS, and AIDSDRUGS which are produced by the National Library of Medicine, to bulletin boards or messaging systems such as Computerized AIDS Information Network (CAIN) produced by the Los Angeles Gay and Lesbian Community Services Center. More recently, a plethora of HIV/AIDS-related information has been made available via the Internet, including the vast resources accessible using the World Wide Web.

SPECIALIZED INFORMATION RESOURCES AND SERVICES

Bibliographies

Information services focusing on HIV/AIDS are supported by various organizations–some being more traditional information providers than others–in varying degrees. One of the earliest information services to be offered concerning HIV/AIDS was the compilation of relevant bibliographies. These specialized resources continue to prove invaluable. The emergence of disease-specific bibliographies may be traced back to the early 1980s. Their appearance paralleled the classification of the constellation of conditions and opportunistic infections associated with the illness as the *acquired immunodeficiency syndrome* and the identification of the *human immunodeficiency virus* as the causative agent of the disease.

In 1983, the National Library of Medicine (NLM) began publishing *Acquired Immunodeficiency Syndrome (AIDS)* as part of its Literature Search Service.[1] (This was the same year that NLM introduced the term "acquired immunodeficiency syndrome" into its controlled vocabulary, *Medical Subject Headings (MeSH)*.) The initial issue in this series was retrospective in nature, and included citations with publication dates back to 1981. This series ceased publication in 1987, and was succeeded by *AIDS Bibliography*.[2] *AIDS Bibliography* contains citations to AIDS-related materials indexed in NLM databases in the preclinical, epidemiologic, diagnostic, and prevention areas.

NLM's *AIDS Bibliography* is one of the most extensive, ongoing, print bibliographies concerning HIV/AIDS. Although it is one of the oldest and broadest in scope of coverage, it is by no means the only published bibliography or, in some instances, the most appropriate. *AIDS Bibliography* is limited to materials indexed for the databases NLM produces, but other bibliographies are not. In addition, other bibliographies such as *AIDS Targeted*

Information Newsletter (A.T.I.N.) include abstracts and/or critical editorial comments. Furthermore, bibliographies focusing on particular areas of interest, disciplines, specialties, and/or subspecialties have been, and continue to be, compiled and published. These subject-specific bibliographies allow for more comprehensive coverage of a particular topic as it relates to HIV/AIDS than their more general counterparts. (For an expanded listing of existing bibliographies, consult one of the information directories mentioned in the previous chapter or consult one of the HIV/AIDS-related electronic databases.)

Newsletters

Another service often provided by organizations working within the AIDS arena that yields an information resource is the production and distribution of newsletters. Newsletters serve as a vital link between individuals directly affected by HIV/AIDS and current information regarding existing programs and services (e.g., legal, medical, nutritional, psychosocial), advances in medical management of HIV/AIDS, drug clinical trials, and current events. Newsletters often contain clinical and/or pharmaceutical information gleaned from the technical literature, restated and summarized in terminology comprehensible to the lay person. In addition, HIV/AIDS newsletters have evolved into recognized sources of information for the health care practitioner as well, particularly where the most recent information concerning drug development and usage is concerned. The value of these nontraditional resources as sources of information may be evidenced in the fact that key traditional information producers such as the National Library of Medicine have begun to selectively index them for inclusion in biomedical databases.

Electronic Resources

The host of electronic sources of information concerning HIV/AIDS currently available varies in form and content from the more common bibliographic databases to the multitude of resources accessible via the Internet. Electronic resources are available online, on disk, in CD-ROM format, and via the Internet. This rich bevy of specialized data sources provides information concerning every aspect of the disease. Electronic resources are produced and used by a variety of individuals and groups including health care professionals, staff members working in AIDS service organizations, information professionals, hospice workers, and individuals directly affected by HIV/AIDS.

Perhaps the most common electronic resources relative to HIV and AIDS are bibliographic databases. These databases typically provide references to the published literature concerning the disease. While most general bibliographic databases contain references to AIDS-related information due to the pervasive nature of the illness–HIV/AIDS is a cross-disciplinary, interdisciplinary, and multidisciplinary topic–there are bibliographic databases devoted solely to HIV/AIDS. The two main disease-specific bibliographic databases are AIDSLINE, produced by the National Library of Medicine in the United States, and AIDS Database, produced by the Bureau of Hygiene and Tropical Diseases in the United Kingdom. Both focus on the biomedical, epidemiologic, health care administration, oncologic, and social and behavioral sciences literature.

An important complement to bibliographic databases are factual databases such as AIDSDRUGS and AIDSTRIALS, both available through the National Library of Medicine, MEDLARS Management Section. (Where bibliographic databases refer the user to published literature for information, factual databases supply the actual information.) AIDSDRUGS and AIDSTRIALS provide access to information compiled and maintained as part of the AIDS Clinical Trials Information Service project. AIDSDRUGS contains information about the agents being tested in clinical trials relative to HIV/AIDS, while AIDSTRIALS includes information about actual clinical trials of agents undergoing investigation for use against acquired immunodeficiency syndrome, HIV infection, and HIV/AIDS-related opportunistic diseases and infections. AIDSDRUGS includes such things as synonyms for the drug name, pharmacological information, and descriptive information. AIDSTRIALS includes such things as the protocol title, drug information, a general description of what disease or infection the drug is being used to treat, clinical trial inclusion/exclusion criteria, whether the trial is open or closed, geographic location of the trial, and the supporting agency.

Another significant factual database is *The AIDS Knowledge Base,* which is produced under the direction of the San Francisco General Hospital AIDS Program. *The AIDS Knowledge Base* is a textbook for treating HIV and AIDS. It includes the full text of more than 300 original chapters and articles concerning most aspects of the human immunodeficiency virus, acquired immunodeficiency syndrome, and related issues, infections, and diseases. (Although *The AIDS Knowledge Base* was initially only available in electronic format, it is now available in print as well.) In addition to these key resources, various other databases exist. These include, but are not limited to, AIDS Information and Education Worldwide, produced by CD Resources, Inc.; Combined Health Information Database (CHID) produced by the U.S. Public Health Service (with contributions from various health-related government education programs including the CDC National AIDS Information and Education Program); and AIDS Compact Library, produced by Paramount Publishing.

In addition to HIV/AIDS-related online, on disk, and CD-ROM databases, a variety of resources are available electronically via the Internet or, in some cases, using dial-up access. Internet resources include electronic bulletin boards, discussion lists, news groups, full-text documents available using file transfer protocol (ftp), and the myriad of hypertext/hypermedia resources accessible using gophers and the World Wide Web. A natural advantage to Internet resources is cost–accessing resources via the Internet generally eliminates long distance telephone charges and connect fees. (Unfortunately not all electronic bulletin boards, databases, and information services are available via the Internet, but require dial-up access using a modem.) With the Internet and an appropriate browser, users can view the Agency for Health Care Policy and Research (AHCPR) guidelines for treating HIV infection; review the most recent epidemiological statistics available from the U.S. Centers for Disease Control and Prevention or the World Health Organization; examine current developments in the basic science of HIV/AIDS; become familiar with various AIDS service organizations and the services they offer; and communicate with other researchers, clinicians, practitioners, educators, caregivers, or individuals directly affected by HIV/AIDS. (See Appendix C for sample Internet resource sites.)

SPECIAL INFORMATION CENTERS AND SERVICES

Due to the impact of HIV disease and AIDS on society, many traditional organizations are offering nontraditional services or expanding existing services into less traditional venues. In addition, this disease has spawned the creation of a variety of community-based centers and/or services in response to the demand for accurate and timely information. One example of this phenomenon–a traditional institution's providing a nontraditional service–was the incorporation of a computerized program in the information services component of the Norman Public Library in Norman, Oklahoma, to help determine whether or not one should be tested for HIV.[3] The program provides general HIV/AIDS information, requests information regarding the user's background where potential risk for infection is concerned, analyzes the response, and prints out its recommendation regarding testing. While many public libraries have developed current awareness information centers or services focusing on HIV/AIDS, few have sought to facilitate the delivery of health care to this degree.

Another example of a library's redefining its boundaries may be evinced in the Department of Veterans Affairs AIDS Information Center located at the San Francisco VA Medical Center. The AIDS Information Center was established in 1989 in response to the growing needs of individuals involved in VA HIV/AIDS education, patient care, and research. The Center functions as an integral component of the VA's National HIV/AIDS Education Initiatives. In addition to the many services the Center supports to facilitate information access and exchange, the *AIDS Information Newsletter*–produced on site and widely distributed–is perhaps the most renowned. The *Newsletter* is recognized as a resource for subject-specific reviews of HIV/AIDS-related issues.

An additional significant example of a contributor to the HIV/AIDS information arena is the Computerized AIDS Information Network (CAIN), a component of the Los Angeles Gay and Lesbian Community Services Center. CAIN resulted from the gay and lesbian community's recognition, early on in the epidemic, of the importance of information. The Network is an electronic communications service that facilitates access to information relevant to the disease. CAIN maintains HIV/AIDS-related databases and provides electronic mail, bulletin board, conference, and opinion poll services.

While many AIDS service organizations and community-based organizations currently include an information center or library facility, few–if any–rival the AIDS Information Network (AIN). The AIN, formerly the AIDS Library of Philadelphia, is the largest HIV/AIDS-specific lending library in the United States designed for public use. It provides comprehensive, current information regarding all aspects of HIV and AIDS to anyone who requests it. The AIN houses a collection of print, electronic, and audiovisual materials; provides referrals; supports a speaker's bureau; provides research assistance; and produces and distributes a newsletter (the *Critical Path AIDS Project* is an AIN program) that serves as a digest of current drug, treatment, and clinical trials information.

Not all specialized information centers or services exist, however, at the community level or stem from more traditional public service organizations or institutions. The National AIDS Clearinghouse (NAC) is an excellent example of a U.S. government information resource created in response to the public demand for information. The NAC operates under a contract from the Centers for Disease Control and Prevention and functions as a centralized source for government-approved information regarding materials, programs, and services relative to HIV and AIDS. The National AIDS Clearinghouse maintains several inhouse databases and electronic resources–including the AIDS Daily Summaries, a directory of organizations, a conference database, an educational materials database, a funding opportunities database, and an electronic bulletin board service–that are accessible to the public via direct connect or by telephoning the NAC for assistance. In addition to being actively involved in outreach, the Clearinghouse facilitates the development of a nationwide interactive network of HIV/AIDS libraries and information services.

As a component of the National AIDS Clearinghouse, the AIDS Clinical Trials Information Service (ACTIS) is a central resource that provides current information on federally and privately sponsored clinical trials for people with HIV and AIDS. This Public Health Service project is provided collaboratively by the Centers for Disease Control and Prevention, the Food and Drug Administration, the National Institute of Allergy and Infectious Diseases, and the National Library of Medicine. The information contained in the ACTIS database may be accessed by telephoning a health specialist at ACTIS, or directly through AIDSDRUGS or AIDSTRIALS.

Another U.S. interagency collaborative effort is the HIV/AIDS Treatment Information Service (ATIS) operating under the

Department of Health and Human Services and supported by the Agency for Health Care Policy and Research, Centers for Disease Control and Prevention, Health Resources and Services Administration, Indian Health Service, National Institutes of Health, and Substance Abuse and Mental Health Services Administration. ATIS is offered through the CDC National AIDS Clearinghouse and provides access to information concerning federally approved treatment guidelines.

The United States is not alone in its efforts to establish centralized government information resources concerning HIV/AIDS. Many countries have established national AIDS hotlines, information lines, information services and centers. *European AIDS Information and Documentation Centers* [4] provides a listing and brief description of HIV/AIDS information centers throughout Europe. Examples of the global expanse of HIV/AIDS-specific information resources include the Federal Centre for AIDS (Canada's Department of National Health and Welfare's first single-disease directorate),[5] the AIDS Archives Project of the AIDS Social History Programme (a component of the London School of Hygiene and Tropical Medicine),[6] and the AIDS Information Exchange Resource Centre at the African Regional Health Education Centre (established as an integral component of the World Health Organization's Global Programme on AIDS).[7]

CONCLUSION

Specialized HIV/AIDS information resources and services have sprung from a recognized need–information is key to efforts devoted to stemming the spread of the epidemic, advancing research and treatment, fostering empathy toward affected individuals, and empowering individuals living with the disease. The demand for information has yielded disease-specific resources, services, and centers that are diverse in nature. As with HIV and

AIDS, these resources are not limited to a particular population, culture, or country. Rather, they may be found existing or operating at various levels throughout the world. Although different in appearance and universal in occurrence, they are bound by the same common thread–HIV/AIDS.

REFERENCES

1. *Acquired Immunodeficiency Syndrome (AIDS)*. Bethesda, MD: U.S. Dept. of Health and Human Services, Public Health Service, National Institutes of Health, 1983-1988. [Continued by AIDS Bibliography.]

2. *AIDS Bibliography*. Bethesda, MD: U.S. Dept. of Health and Human Services, Public Health Service, National Institutes of Health, National Library of Medicine, Reference Section, 1988– .

3. HIV test available in: Norman PL. Computer program allows users to privately check HIV potential. *Library Journal*. 117:26;1992 Mar 1.

4. Dresslar S, Hommes M (eds.). *European AIDS Information and Documentation Centers*. Berlin: AIDS-Zentrum im Bundesgesundheitsamt, 1992.

5. Cohen L. The Federal Centre for AIDS: working against a plague mentality. *CMAJ–Canadian Medical Association Journal*. 138(9):839-840,1988 May 1.

6. Foster J. *AIDS Archives in the UK*. London: London School of Hygiene and Tropical Medicine, 1990.

7. Olaseha IO; Adeniyi JD. The birth of the WHO/GPA Regional AIDS Information Exchange Resource Centre; African Regional Health Education Centre, University of Ibadan, Nigeria. *Hygie*. 10(4):49-50, 1991.

Chapter 4

Information Networking and Partnerships

RESOURCE SHARING

Resource sharing is not a new concept. However, the variety of individuals, institutions, and organizations working within the AIDS arena have limited the extent of information networking in this area. As the epidemic spreads, the impetus for sharing of existing resources grows. Due to the diverse nature of HIV/AIDS-related information and consumers of that information, it simply is not possible for a single institution or organization to be the sole, comprehensive resource for all potential health information consumers.

NETWORKING AND PARTNERSHIPS

Information networks have evolved along with technological advances, expanding computing capabilities, and the changing nature of information consumers. Historically, information networks typically have been mutually beneficial contractual agreements–verbal or written, formal or informal–between two or more departments, libraries, institutions, or organizations to share information resources. At baseline, information networking involved the physical sharing of print resources and possibly referral to another, or more appropriate, information provider. In many ways, this model is similar in nature to a series of partnerships. Most often, participants have been libraries with a common charter, goal, or interest (e.g., located in the same geographic region, belonging to the same parent organization or institution, and sharing similar collection focuses). At this level, networks benefit directly participating members and indirectly information consumers. This model, of course, assumes traditional modes of information production and consumption. Primary focus is placed on the traditional information repository (i.e., the library) rather than the individual or nontraditional information provider. Networks of this type have fostered a library-centered approach to information access.

However, information networking and partnerships have evolved over time to reflect the current focus on outreach and end-user access to information. (Traditional information networks continue to exist, of course, for support purposes. The underlying philosophy has simply been expanded, using modern technology, to serve and complement the current status of information creators, consumers, and disseminators.) HIV/AIDS may be seen as a model that exemplifies the changing nature of the health information creator, consumer, and disseminator, and as an illustration of the evolution of information networks and partnerships.

Many of the electronic information resources discussed in the previous chapter could easily be included within the guise of networking and partnerships. The vast majority of HIV/AIDS specialized information resources and services are the result of some form of a partnership or have evolved from an information network in response to consumer needs. Most databases and electronic resources may be accessed directly, and function as an integral component of the growing global HIV/AIDS information network. Included here, however, are examples of networking and partnerships that have not yet been discussed.

The Southeast Florida AIDS Information Network

The Southeast Florida AIDS Information Network (SEFAIN)[1] is a relatively early example of a specialized information system designed to function as a community outreach project. SEFAIN was designed at the Louis Calder Memorial Library, University of Miami School of Medicine, to facilitate electronic information access to local AIDS service providers. The project was funded by the National Library of Medicine in 1990 to serve as a prototype for the tri-county Florida area. For this undertaking, bibliographic records for materials related to HIV/AIDS housed in the various libraries within the University of Miami were loaded into the online public access catalog. In addition, an alternate database was created containing information about current research studies underway in the southeast Florida area as well as directory information concerning local AIDS service providers. SEFAIN serves as a model for providing networked access to information resources within a traditional library setting.

The Dallas AIDS Resource Center

Perhaps one of the most unique examples of networking and partnerships resulting from the information demands created by HIV/AIDS exists at the AIDS Resource Center in Dallas, Texas. The Center opened its library and historic archives to the public in 1994 as part of a physical facility renovation, but with limited funding for library resources. Through networking and the formation of a series of partnerships, however, the library has evolved into an invaluable community information resource. A planned giving program has been coordinated with a local bookstore to assist with collection development. Bookstore patrons purchase books for the library's collection based on need as established by the librarian–somewhat similar in nature to a bridal gift registry. In addition, the bookstore sponsors an authors' speakers' bureau with a portion of the lectures being given at the AIDS Resource Center. To assist further with collection development, primarily where scientific and biomedical texts are concerned, the librarian has coordinated a planned giving program through a major book vendor. In conjunction with a vendor representative, the librarian performs a periodic mailing to local health care practitioners requesting needed items, which are available through the vendor. Collection development is coordinated with the local branch of the public library so as not to duplicate effort. Moreover, an arrangement has been made establishing a referral service between the Center's library and the public library to ensure adequate reference coverage. Through a creative approach, the library has established itself as a hub within the community's HIV/AIDS information network.

The Gay Men's Health Crisis and the New York Public Library

Another nontraditional partnership resulting from HIV/AIDS is the one that has been formed between the Gay Men's Health Crisis (GMHC) and the New York Public Library. GMHC is one of the largest AIDS service organizations in the United States. In addition to supporting a variety of information-related services, the Gay Men's Health Crisis produces a newsletter–*Treatment Issues*–that is widely recognized as an authoritative resource regarding current therapeutic efforts. As a significant contributor to the body of information concerning the epidemic, GMHC fills an important archival function where HIV and AIDS are concerned. The New York Public Library recognized the value of the continued historical collection of materials concerning the pandemic, and arranged to house the archives of the Gay Men's Health Crisis.

The National Library of Medicine

The importance of information networks and nontraditional partnerships has been widely recognized, so much so that the National Library of Medicine (NLM) began funding a series of projects in this vein in 1994. The focus of the NLM-funded projects is to facilitate information access at the community level. Collaborative efforts are encouraged by NLM between community-based organizations, AIDS service providers, public libraries, health sciences libraries, and other concerned organizations or institutions. The ultimate goal is to provide timely, accurate HIV/AIDS-related information when and where it is needed.

CONCLUSION

Providing universal access to HIV/AIDS-related information–riddled with complexities and continuously increasing in volume–necessitates the creation of networks and the formation of partnerships. HIV/AIDS information networks and partnerships are as diverse in nature as the creators and consumers of HIV/AIDS-related information. In some instances, the players and scenario are quite traditional. In what seems to be more common, however, the enabling body that facilitates HIV/AIDS-related information access is the result of a nontraditional partnership forged out of demand.

REFERENCE

1. Burrows S, Perry MJ, Tylman VT, Lemkau HL. The Southeast Florida AIDS Information Network: A community outreach, specialized information system. *Medical Reference Services Quarterly.* 13(1): 1-18, 1994.

Chapter 5

Looking Beyond Existing Resources and Services

RELATIVE INFANCY AND THE INITIATION OF AN INFORMATION INFRASTRUCTURE

The HIV/AIDS epidemic is more than ten years old. However, programs designed to provide information to an HIV-affected population are, for the most part, in the infancy stage. The confluence of roles among information creators, providers, and seekers within the AIDS arena has highlighted many of the flaws in the existing information delivery system, and has afforded the opportunity to improve significantly upon that structure by recognizing and revising the process.[1] Through research designed to identify and fill information voids, the encouragement of collaborative efforts, the establishment of enhanced networks, and the creation of aggressive and creative outreach programs, the effective provision of AIDS-related information and services to HIV-infected individuals, those at risk for infection, and the affected community can be achieved. However, this has yet to be realized fully.

CURRENT BARRIERS AND IMPEDIMENTS

While much has been done to bridge the communications gap within the AIDS arena and to facilitate access to existing information, barriers and impediments continue to exist. The very nature of the information, the stigma associated with the disease, and societal perceptions of the epidemic's affiliation with the population most affected initially in the United States all serve to deter effective dissemination of the body of knowledge concerning HIV/AIDS, as well as deter the creation and utilization of shared resources.

The body of information concerning this disease is voluminous and continues to grow at an alarming rate. Electronic resources such as the AIDS-related bibliographic databases have been developed to facilitate information access, but no one is comprehensive. HIV/AIDS-related information spans multiple disciplines, thus requiring the use of various resources in order to obtain all relevant information. This means that the information consumer must be aware of those resources and be familiar with the variety of controlled vocabularies used for indexing purposes as well as the different interfaces and command languages employed within each system. A better means to organize the body of knowledge and effectively disseminate HIV/AIDS information needs to be developed.

In addition to the amount of information that currently exists concerning HIV/AIDS, the subject matter itself has created obstacles to the effective dissemination of information. Content of the information has often been controversial, thus limiting its ready availability. Societal perceptions of HIV and AIDS-related information directly affects the key role that information plays where this disease is concerned.

Efforts to coordinate communication among HIV/AIDS information providers have been, at best, limited. HIV/AIDS-related information is produced and supplied at a variety of levels by numerous individuals, institutions, and organizations throughout the world. Exchange of information among HIV/AIDS information providers occurs all too often in a haphazard fashion. A single, effective, international communication forum targeting HIV/AIDS information providers simply does not currently exist.

While specialized resources and services have begun to be developed and creative partnerships formed, availability and accessibility of HIV/AIDS-related information remain limited. Obstacles remain. Necessity, however, demands the continued development of a creative information infrastructure that supports the efficacious delivery of information concerning HIV and AIDS.

CONCLUSION

Information plays a key role within the AIDS pandemic. It forms the basis for education, and education is currently the only means by which to slow the spread of HIV infection. Information is a central component in furthering the medical management of the disease. Information in the form of books, audio tapes, videos, and electronic resources functions as a form of entertainment and support to those already infected. While HIV/AIDS data may not always be easily accessible and barriers to services for HIV-infected individuals may exist, the importance of the provision of information cannot be overemphasized. This is a modern-day epidemic that affects all.

REFERENCE

1. Ginn DS. The development of specialized biomedical information. *Library Trends*. 42(1):180-195, 1993.

Appendix A

Case Definitions of AIDS

This appendix contains the selective text of case definitions of AIDS as they have appeared in the published literature (see the original articles for the complete text). Revisions mirror increased understanding of the illness, and variations reflect the difficulties associated with defining the disease.

PART I: 1993 EXPANSION OF THE CDC SURVEILLANCE CASE DEFINITION FOR AIDS AMONG ADOLESCENTS AND ADULTS[1]

In 1991, CDC, in collaboration with the Council of State and Territorial Epidemiologists (CSTE), proposed an expansion of the AIDS surveillance case definition. This proposal was made available for public comment in November 1991 and was discussed at an open meeting on September 2, 1992. Based on information presented and reviewed during the public comment period and at the open meeting, CDC, in collaboration with CSTE, expanded the AIDS surveillance case definition to include all HIV-infected persons with CD4+ T-lymphocyte counts of <200 cells/cubic millimeter or a CD4+ percentage of <14. In addition to retaining the 23 clinical conditions in the previous AIDS surveillance definition, the expanded definition includes pulmonary tuberculosis (TB), recurrent pneumonia, and invasive cervical cancer. This expanded definition requires laboratory confirmation of HIV infection in persons with a CD4+ T-lymphocyte count of <200 cells/cubic millimeter or with one of the added clinical conditions. This expanded definition for reporting cases to CDC became effective January 1, 1993.

In the revised HIV classification system, persons in subcategories A3, B3, and C3 meet the immunologic criteria of the surveillance case definition, and those persons with conditions in subcategories C1, C2, and C3 meet the clinical criteria for surveillance purposes (see Appendix B, Part I: 1993 CDC Revised HIV Classification System for Adolescents and Adults). A, B, and C refer to 1.A, 1.B, and 1.C on the following pages. The numbers 1, 2, and 3 refer to the CD4+ T-cell categories depicted in Table 1A. The alphabetic are the conditions and the numeric are the CD4+ T-lymphocyte categories.

*I.A. Equivalences for Absolute Numbers of CD4+ T-lymphocytes and CD4+ Percentage**

CD4+ T-cell category	CD4+ T-cells/cubic millimeter	CD4+ percentage (%)
(1)	≥500	≥29
(2)	200-499	14-28
(3)	<200	<14

I.B. Conditions Included in the 1993 AIDS Surveillance Case Definition

– Candidiasis of bronchi, trachea, or lungs
– Candidiasis, esophageal
– Cervical cancer, invasive**
– Coccidioidomycosis, disseminated or extrapulmonary
– Cryptococcosis, extrapulmonary

*The percentage of lymphocytes that are CD4+ T-cells.

**Added in the 1993 expansion of the AIDS surveillance case definition.

– Cryptosporidiosis, chronic intestinal (>1 month's duration)
– Cytomegalovirus disease (other than liver, spleen, or nodes)
– Cytomegalovirus retinitis (with loss of vision)
– Encephalopathy, HIV-related
– Herpes simplex: chronic ulcer(s) (>1 month's duration); or bronchitis, pneumonitis, or esophagitis
– Histoplasmosis, disseminated or extrapulmonary
– Isosporiasis, chronic intestinal (>1 month's duration)
– Kaposi's sarcoma
– Lymphoma, Burkitt's (or equivalent term)
– Lymphoma, immunoblastic (or equivalent term)
– Lymphoma, primary, of brain
– *Mycobacterium avium* complex or *M. kansasii,* disseminated or extrapulmonary
– *Mycobacterium tuberculosis,* any site (pulmonary** or extrapulmonary)
– *Mycobacterium,* other species or unidentified species, disseminated or exptrapulmonary
– *Pneumocystis carinii* pneumonia
– Pneumonia, recurrent**
– Progressive multifocal leukoencephalopathy
– *Salmonella* septicemia, recurrent
– Toxoplasmosis of brain
– Wasting syndrome due to HIV

I.C. Definitive Diagnostic Methods for Diseases Indicative of AIDS

Diseases	Diagnostic Methods
Cryptosporidiosis Isosporiasis Kaposi's sarcoma	Microscopy (histology or cytology)

**Added in the 1993 expansion of the AIDS surveillance case definition.

Lymphoma *Pneumocystis carinii* pneumonia Progressive multifocal leukoencephalopathy Toxoplasmosis Cervical cancer	
Candidiasis	Gross inspection by endoscopy or autopsy or by microscopy (histology or cytology) on a specimen obtained directly from the tissues affected (including scraping from the mucosal surface), not from a culture
Coccidioidomycosis Cryptococcosis Cytomegalovirus Herpes simplex virus Histoplasmosis	Microscopy (histology or cytology), culture, or detection of antigen in a specimen obtained directly from the tissues affected or a fluid from those tissues
Tuberculosis Other mycobacteriosis Salmonellosis	Culture
HIV encephalopathy (dementia)	Clinical findings of disabling cognitive or motor dysfunction interfering with occupation or activities of daily living, progressing over weeks to months, in the absence of a concurrent illness or condition other than HIV infection that could explain the findings. Methods to rule out such concurrent illness and conditions must include cerebrospinal fluid examina-

	tion and either brain imaging (computed tomography or magnetic resonance) or autopsy.
HIV wasting syndrome	Findings of profound involuntary weight loss of >10 percent of baseline body weight plus either chronic diarrhea (at least two loose stools per day for $\geq$30 days), or chronic weakness and documented fever (for $\geq$30 days, intermittent or constant) in the absence of a concurrent illness or condition other than HIV infection that could explain the findings (e.g., cancer, tuberculosis, cryptosporidiosis, or other specific enteritis).
Pneumonia, recurrent	Recurrent (more than one episode in a one-year period), acute (new x-ray evidence not present earlier) pneumonia diagnosed by both: (a) culture (or other organism-specific diagnostic method) obtained from a clinically reliable specimen of a pathogen that typically causes pneumonia (other than *Pneumocystis carinii* or *Mycobacterium tuberculosis*), and (b) radiologic evidence of pneumonia; cases that do not have laboratory confirmation of a causative organism for one of the episodes of pneumonia will be considered to be presumptively diagnosed.

I.D. Suggested Guidelines for Presumptive Diagnosis of Disease Indicative of AIDS

Diseases	Presumptive Criteria
Candidiasis of esophagus	a. Recent onset of retrosternal pain on swallowing; AND b. Oral candidiasis diagnosed by the gross appearance of white patches or plaques on an erythematous base or by the microscopic appearance of fungal mycelial filaments from a noncultured specimen scraped from the oral mucosa.
Cytomegalovirus retinits	A characteristic appearance on serial ophthalmoscopic examinations (e.g., discrete patches of retinal whitening with distinct borders, spreading in a centrifugal manner along the paths of blood vessels, progressing over several months, and frequently associated with retinal vasculitis, hemorrhage, and necrosis). Resolution of active disease leaves retinal scarring and atrophy with retinal pigment epithelial mottling.
Mycobacteriosis	Microscopy of a specimen from stool or normally sterile body fluids or tissue from a site other than lungs, skin, or cervical or hilar lymph nodes that shows acid-fast bacilli of a species not identified by culture.
Kaposi's sarcoma	A characteristic gross appearance of an erythematous or violaceous plaque-

	like lesion on skin or mucous membrane. (Note: Presumptive diagnosis of Kaposi's sarcoma should not be made by clinicians who have seen few cases of it.)
Pneumocystis carinii pneumonia	a. A history of dyspnea on exertion or nonproductive cough of recent onset (within the past three months); AND b. Chest x-ray evidence of diffuse bilateral interstitial infiltrates or evidence by gallium scan of diffuse bilateral pulmonary disease; AND c. Arterial blood gas analysis showing an arterial Po_2 of <70 mm Hg or a low respiratory diffusing capacity (<80 percent of predicted values) or an increase in the alveolar-arterial oxygen tension gradient; AND d. No evidence of a bacterial pneumonia.
Pneumonia, recurrent	Recurrent (more than one episode in a one-year period), acute (new symptoms, signs, or x-ray evidence not present earlier) pneumonia diagnosed on clinical or radiologic grounds by the patient's physician.
Toxoplasmosis of brain	a. Recent onset of a focal neurologic abnormality consistent with intracranial disease or a reduced level of consciousness; AND b. Evidence by brain imaging (computed tomography or nuclear magnetic resonance) of a lesion having a

	mass effect or the radiographic appearance of which is enhance by injection of contrast medium; AND c. Serum antibody to toxoplasmosis or successful response to therapy for toxoplasmosis.
Tuberculosis, pulmonary	When bacteriologic confirmation is not available, other reports may be considered to be verified cases of pulmonary tuberculosis if the criteria of the Division of Tuberculosis Elimination, National Center for Prevention Services, CDC, are used. The criteria in use as of January 1, 1993, are available in *MMWR* 1990; 39(No. RR-13): 39-40.

PART II: 1987 REVISION OF THE CDC SURVEILLANCE CASE DEFINITION FOR AIDS[2]

Introduction

The following revised case definition for surveillance of acquired immunodeficiency syndrome (AIDS) was developed by CDC in collaboration with public health and clinical specialists. The Council of State and Territorial Epidemiologists (CSTE) has officially recommended adoption of the revised definition for national reporting of AIDS. The objectives of the revision are (a) to track more effectively the severe disabling morbidity associated with infection with human immunodeficiency virus (HIV) (including HIV-1 and HIV-2); (b) to simplify reporting of

AIDS cases; (c) to increase the sensitivity and specificity of the definition through greater diagnostic application of laboratory evidence for HIV infection; and (d) to be consistent with current diagnostic practice, which in some cases includes presumptive, i.e., without confirmatory laboratory evidence, diagnosis of AIDS-indicative diseases (e.g., *Pneumocystis carinii* pneumonia, Kaposi's sarcoma).

The definition is organized into three sections that depend on the status of laboratory evidence of HIV infection (e.g., HIV antibody) (see Table 1). The major proposed changes apply to patients with laboratory evidence for HIV infection: (a) inclusion of HIV encephalopathy, HIV wasting syndrome, and a broader range of specific AIDS-indicative diseases (Table 1, 2.A.); (b) inclusion of AIDS patients whose indicator diseases are diagnosed presumptively (Table 1, 2.B.); and (c) elimination of exclusions due to other causes of immunodeficiency (Table 1, 1.A.).

Application of the definition for children differs from that for adults in two ways. First, multiple or recurrent serious bacterial infections and lymphoid interstitial pneumonia/pulmonary lymphoid hyperplasia are accepted as indicative of AIDS among children but not among adults. Second, for children >15 months of age whose mothers are thought to have had HIV infection during the child's perinatal period, the laboratory criteria for HIV infection are more stringent, since the presence of HIV antibody in the child is, by itself, insufficient evidence for HIV infection because of the persistence of passively acquired maternal antibodies >15 months after birth.

The initiation of the actual reporting of cases that meet the new definition is targeted for September 1, 1987. CSTE has recommended retrospective application of the revised definition to patients already reported to health departments. The new definition is presented in Table 1.

Table 1. 1987 Revision of Case Definition for AIDS for Surveillance Purposes

For national reporting, a case of AIDS is defined as an illness characterized by one or more of the following "indicator" diseases, depending on the status of laboratory evidence of HIV infection, as shown below.

1. Without Laboratory Evidence Regarding HIV Infection

If laboratory tests for HIV were not performed or gave inconclusive results (see Appendix A, Part II.A.) and the patient had no other cause of immunodeficiency listed in 1.A. below, then any disease listed in 1.B. below indicates AIDS if it was diagnosed by a definitive method (see Appendix A, Part II.B.).

1.A. Causes of immunodeficiency that disqualify disease as indicators of AIDS in the absence of laboratory evidence for HIV infection:

1. high-dose or long-term systemic corticosteroid therapy or other immunosuppressive/cytotoxic therapy < 3 months before the onset of the indicator disease;
2. any of the following disease diagnosed < 3 months after diagnosis of the indicator disease: Hodgkin's disease, non-Hodgkin's lymphoma (other than primary brain lymphoma), lymphocytic leukemia, multiple myeloma, any other cancer of lymphoreticular or histiocytic tissue, or angioimmunoblastic lymphadenopathy;
3. a genetic (congenital) immunodeficiency syndrome or an acquired immunodeficiency syndrome atypical of HIV infection, such as one involving hypogammaglobulinemia.

1.B. Indicator diseases diagnosed definitively (see Appendix A, Part II.B.):

1. candidiasis of the esophagus, trachea, bronchi, or lungs;
2. cryptococcosis, extrapulmonary;
3. cryptosporidiosis with diarrhea persisting >1 month;
4. cytomegalovirus disease of an organ other than liver, spleen, or lymph nodes in a patient >1 month of age;
5. herpes simplex virus infection causing a mucocutaneous ulcer that persists longer than one month; or bronchitis, pneumonitis, or esophagitis for any duration affecting a patient >1 month of age;
6. Kaposi's sarcoma affecting a patient >60 years of age;
7. lymphoma of the brain (primary) affecting a patient >60 years of age;
8. lymphoid interstitial pneumonia and/or pulmonary lymphoid hyperplasia (LIP/PLH complex) affecting a child <13 years of age;
9. *Mycobacterium avium* complex or *M. kansasii* disease, disseminated (at a site other than or in addition to lungs, skin, or cervical or hilar lymph nodes);

10. *Pneumocystis carinii* pneumonia;
11. progressive multifocal leukoencephalopathy;
12. toxoplasmosis of the brain affecting a patient >1 month of age.

2. With Laboratory Evidence for HIV Infection

Regardless of the presence of other causes of immunodeficiency (1.A. above), in the presence of laboratory evidence for HIV infection (see Appendix A, Part II.B.), any disease listed above (1.B.) or below (2.A. or 2.B.) indicates a diagnosis of AIDS.

2.A. Indicator diseases diagnosed definitively (see Appendix A, Part II.B.):

1. bacterial infections, multiple or recurrent (any combination of at least two within a two-year period), of the following types affecting a child <13 years of age:

   septicemia, pneumonia, meningitis, bone or going infection, or abscess of an internal organ or body cavity (excluding otitis media or superficial skin or mucosal abscesses), caused by *Haemophilus, Streptococcus* (including pneumococcus), or other pyogenic bacteria;

2. coccidioidomycosis, disseminated (at a site other than or in addition to lungs or cervical or hilar lymph nodes);
3. HIV encephalopathy (also called "HIV dementia," "AIDS dementia," or "subacute encephalitis due to HIV") (see Appendix A, Part II.B. for description);
4. histoplasmosis, disseminated (at a site other than or in addition to lungs or cervical or hilar lymph nodes);
5. isosporiasis with diarrhea persisting >1 month;
6. Kaposi's sarcoma at any age;
7. lymphoma of the brain (primary) at any age;
8. other non-Hodgkin's lymphoma of B-cell or unknown immunologic phenotype and the following histologic types:
   a. small noncleaved lymphoma (either Burkitt or non-Burkitt type) (see Appendix A, Part II.D. for equivalent terms and numeric codes used in the *International Classification of Diseases,* Ninth Revision, Clinical Modification);
   b. immunoblastic sarcoma (equivalent to any of the following, although not necessarily all in combination: immunoblastic lymphoma, large-cell lymphoma, diffuse histiocytic lymphoma, diffuse undifferentiated lymphoma, or high-grade lymphoma) (see Appendix A, Part II.D. for equivalent terms and numeric codes used in the *International Classification of Diseases,* Ninth Revision, Clinical Modification);

Note: Lymphomas are not included here if they are of T-cell immunologic phenotype or their histologic type is not described or is described as "lymphocytic," "lymphoblastic," "small cleaved," or "plasmacytoid lymphocytic."

9. any mycobacterial disease caused by mycobacteria other than *M. tuberculosis,* disseminated (at a site other than or in addition to lungs, skin, or cervical or hilar lymph nodes);
10. disease caused by *M. tuberculosis,* extrapulmonary (involving at least one site outside the lungs, regardless of whether there is concurrent pulmonary involvement);
11. *Salmonella* (nontyphoid) septicemia, recurrent;
12. HIV wasting syndrome (emaciation, "slim disease") (see Appendix A, Part II.B. for description).

2.B. Indicator disease diagnosed presumptively (by a method other than those in Appendix A, Part II.B.):

Note: Given the seriousness of diseases indicative of AIDS, it is generally important to diagnose them definitively, especially when therapy that would be used may have serious side effects or when definitive diagnosis is needed for eligibility for antiretroviral therapy. Nonetheless, in some situations, a patient's condition will not permit the performance of definitive tests. In other situations, accepted clinical practice may be to diagnose presumptively based on the presence of characteristic clinical and laboratory abnormalities. Guidelines for presumptive diagnoses are suggested in Appendix A, Part II.C.

1. candidiasis of the esophagus;
2. cytomegalovirus retinitis with loss of vision;
3. Kaposi's sarcoma;
4. lymphoid interstitial pneumonia and/or pulmonary lymphoid hyperplasia (LIP/PLH complex) affecting a child <13 years of age;
5. mycobacterial disease (acid-fast bacilli with species not identified by culture), disseminated (involving at least one site other than or in addition to lungs, skin, or cervical or hilar lymph nodes);
6. *Pneumocystis carinii* pneumonia;
7. toxoplasmosis of the brain affecting a patient >1 month of age.

3. With Laboratory Evidence Against HIV Infection

With laboratory test results negative for HIV infection (see Appendix A, Part II.A.), a diagnosis of AIDS for surveillance purposes is ruled out *unless*:

3.A. all the other causes of immunodeficiency listed above in section 1.A. are excluded; AND

3.B. the patient has had either:

1. *Pneumocystis carinii* pneumonia diagnosed by a definitive method (see Appendix A, Part II.B.); OR

2.a. any of the other disease indicative of AIDS listed above in section 1.B. diagnosed by a definitive method (*See* Appendix A, Part II.B.); AND

b. a T-helper/inducer (CD4) lymphocyte count <400/mm.

II.A. Laboratory Evidence For or Against HIV Infection

1. For Infection:

When a patient has disease consistent with AIDS:

a. a serum specimen from a patient ≥15 months of age, or from a child <15 months of age whose mother is not thought to have had HIV infection during the child's perinatal period, that is repeatedly reactive for HIV antibody by a screening test (e.g., enzyme-linked immunosorbent assay [ELISA]), as long as subsequent HIV-antibody tests (e.g., Western blot, immunofluorescence assay), if done, are positive; **OR**

b. a serum specimen from a child <15 months of age, whose mother is thought to have had HIV infection during the child's perinatal period, that is repeatedly reactive for HIV antibody by a screening test (e.g., ELISA), plus increased serum immunoglobulin levels and at least one of the following abnormal immunologic test results: reduced absolute lymphocyte count, depressed CD4 (T-helper) lymphocyte count, or decreased CD4/CD8 (helper/suppressor) ration, as long as subsequent antibody tests (e.g., Western blot, immunofluorescence assay), if done, are positive; **OR**

c. a positive test for HIV serum antigen; **OR**

d. a positive HIV culture confirmed by both reverse transcriptase detection and a specific HIV-antigen test or in situ hybridization suing a nucleic acid probe; **OR**

e. a positive result on any other highly specific test for HIV (e.g., nucleic acid probe or peripheral blood lymphocytes).

2. Against Infection:

A nonreactive screening test for serum antibody to HIV (e.g., ELISA) without a reactive or positive result on any other test for HIV infection (e.g., antibody, antigen, culture), if done.

3. Inconclusive (Neither For nor Against Infection):

a. a repeatedly reactive screening test for serum antibody to HIV (e.g., ELISA) followed by a negative or inconclusive supplemental test (e.g., Western blot, immunofluorescence assay) without a positive HIV culture or serum antigen test, if done; **OR**
b. a serum specimen from a child <15 months of age, whose mother is thought to have had HIV infection during the child's perinatal period, that is repeatedly reactive for HIV antibody by a screening test, even if positive by a supplemental test, without additional evidence for immunodeficiency as described above (in 1.b.) and without a positive HIV culture or serum antigen test, if done.

II.B. Definitive Diagnostic Methods for Diseases Indicative of AIDS

• Microscopy (histology or cytology):

cryptosporidiosis
cytomegalovirus
isosporiasis
Kaposi's sarcoma
lymphoma
lymphoid pneumonia or hyperplasia
Pneumocystis carinii pneumonia
progressive multifocal leukoencephalopathy
toxoplasmosis

- Gross inspection by endoscopy or autopsy or by microscopy (histology or cytology) on a specimen obtained directly from the tissues affected (including scrapings from the mucosal surface), not from a culture:

    candidiasis

- Microscopy (histology or cytology), culture, or detection of antigen in a specimen obtained directly from the tissues affected or a fluid from those tissues:

    coccidioidomycosis
    cryptococcosis
    herpes simplex virus
    histoplasmosis

- Culture:

    tuberculosis
    other mycobacteriosis
    salmonellosis
    other bacterial infection

- Clinical findings of disabling cognitive and/or motor dysfunction interfering with occupation or activities of daily living, or loss of behavioral developmental milestones affecting a child, progressing over weeks to months, in the absence of a concurrent illness or condition other than HIV infection that could explain the findings. Methods to rule out such concurrent illnesses and conditions must include cerebrospinal fluid examination and either brain imaging (computed tomography or magnetic resonance) or autopsy:

    HIV encephalopathy (dementia)*

- Findings of profound involuntary weight loss >10 percent of baseline body weight plus either chronic diarrhea (at least two

---

*For HIV encephalopathy and HIV wasting syndrome, the methods of diagnosis described here are not truly definitive, but are sufficiently rigorous for surveillance purposes.

loose stools per day for $\geq$30 days) or chronic weakness and documented fever (for $\geq$30 days, intermittent or constant) in the absence of a concurrent illness or condition other than HIV infection that could explain the findings (e.g., cancer, tuberculosis, cryptosporidiosis, or other specific enteritis):

HIV wasting syndrome*

II.C. Suggested Guidelines for Presumptive Diagnosis of Diseases Indicative of AIDS

Diseases	**Presumptive Diagnostic Criteria**
candidiasis of esophagus	a. recent onset of retrosternal pain on swallowing; **AND** b. oral candidiasis diagnosed by the gross appearance of white patches or plaques on an erythematous base or by the microscopic appearance of fungal mycelial filaments in an uncultured specimen scraped from the oral mucosa
cytomegalovirus retinitis	a characteristic appearance on serial ophthalmoscopic examinations (e.g., discrete patches of retinal whitening with distinct borders, spreading in a centrifugal manner, following blood vessels, progressing over several months, frequently associated with retinal vasculitis, hemorrhage, and necrosis). Resolution of active disease leaves retinal scarring and atrophy with retinal pigment epithelial mottling.

*For HIV encephalopathy and HIV wasting syndrome, the methods of diagnosis described here are not truly definitive, but are sufficiently rigorous for surveillance purposes.

mycobacteriosis	microscopy of a specimen from stool or normally sterile body fluids or tissue from a site other than lungs, skin, or cervical or hilar lymph nodes, showing acid-fast bacilli of a species not identified by culture
Kaposi's sarcoma	a characteristic gross appearance of an erythematous or violaceous plaque-like lesion on skin or mucous membranae (**Note:** Presumptive diagnosis of Kaposi's sarcoma should not be made by clinicians who have seen few cases of it.)
lymphoid interstitial pneumonia	bilateral reticulonodular interstitial pulmonary infiltrates present on chest x-ray for ≥ 2 months with no pathogen identified and no response to antibiotic treatment
Pneumocystis carinii pneumonia	a. a history of dyspnea on exertion or nonproductive cough of recent onset (within the past three months); **AND** b. chest x-ray evidence of diffuse bilateral interstitial infiltrates or gallium scan evidence of diffuse bilateral pulmonary disease; **AND** c. arterial blood gas analysis showing an arterial Po_2 of <70 mm Hg or a low respiratory diffusing capacity (<80 percent of predicted values) or an increase in the alveolar-arterial oxygen tension gradient; **AND** d. no evidence of a bacterial pneumonia

toxoplasmosis of the brain	a. recent onset of a focal neurologic abnormality consistent with intracranial disease or a reduced level of consciousness; **AND** b. brain imaging evidence of a lesion having a mass effect (on computed tomography or nuclear magnetic resonance) or the radiographic appearance of which is enhanced by injection of contrast medium; **AND** c. serum antibody to toxoplasmosis or successful response to therapy for toxoplasmosis

II.D. Equivalent Terms and International Classification of Disease (ICD) Codes for AIDS-Indicative Lymphomas

The following terms and codes describe lymphomas indicative of AIDS in patients with antibody evidence for HIV infection. (See AIDS case definition: Table 1, 2.A.8.) Many of these terms are obsolete or equivalent to one another.

ICD-9-CM (1978)

Codes	Terms
200.0	**Reticulosarcoma** lymphoma (malignant): histiocytic (diffuse) reticulum cell sarcoma: pleomorphic cell type or not otherwise specified
200.2	**Burkitt's tumor or lymphoma** malignant lymphoma, Burkitt's type

ICD-O (Oncologic Histologic Types 1976)

Codes	Terms
9600/3	**Malignant lymphoma, undifferentiated cell type**
	non-Burkitt's or not otherwise specified
9601/3	**Malignant lymphoma, stem cell type**
	stem cell lymphoma
9612/3	**Malignant lymphoma, immunoblastic type**
	immunoblastic sarcoma, immunoblastic lymphoma, or immunoblastic lymphosarcoma
9632/3	**Malignant lymphoma, centroblastic type**
	diffuse or not otherwise specified, or germinoblastic sarcoma: diffuse or not otherwise specified
9633/3	**Malignant lymphoma, follicular center cell, non-cleaved**
	diffuse or not otherwise specified
9640/3	**Reticulosarcoma, not otherwise specified**
	malignant lymphoma, histiocytic: diffuse or not otherwise specified reticulum cell sarcoma, not otherwise specified malignant lymphoma, reticulum cell type
9641/3	**Reticulosarcoma, pleomorphic cell type**
	malignant lymphoma, histiocytic, pleomorphic cell type reticulum cell sarcoma, pleomorphic cell type
9750/3	**Burkitt's lymphoma, or Burkitt's tumor**
	malignant lymphoma, undifferentiated, Burkitt's type malignant lymphoma, lymphoblastic, Burkitt's type

PART III: 1985 REVISION OF THE CASE DEFINITION OF ACQUIRED IMMUNODEFICIENCY SYNDROME FOR NATIONAL REPORTING–UNITED STATES[3]

Patients with illnesses that, in retrospect, were manifestations of acquired immunodeficiency syndrome (AIDS) were first described in the summer of 1981.[4,5] A case definition of AIDS for national reporting was first published in *MMWR* in September 1982.[6,7] Since then, the definition has undergone minor revisions in the list of diseases used as indicators of underlying cellular immunodeficiency.[8-11]

Since the 1982 definition was published, human T-cell lymphotropic virus type III/lymphadenopathy-associated virus (HTLV-III/LAV) has been recognized as the cause of AIDS. The clinical manifestations of HTLV-III/LAV infection may be directly attributable to infection with this virus or the result of secondary conditions occurring as a consequence of immune dysfunction caused by the underlying infection with HTLV-III/LAV. The range of manifestations may include none, nonspecific signs and symptoms of illness, autoimmune and neurologic disorders, a variety of opportunistic infections, and several types of malignancy. AIDS was defined for national reporting before its etiology was known, and has encompassed only certain secondary conditions that reliably reflected the presence of a severe immune dysfunction. Current laboratory tests to detect HTLV-III/LAV antibody make it possible to include additional serious conditions in the syndrome, as well as to further improve the specificity of the definition used for reporting cases.

The current case definition of AIDS has provided useful data on disease trends because it is precise, consistently interpreted, and highly specific. Other manifestations of HTLV-III/LAV infections than those currently proposed to be reported are less specific and less likely to be consistently reported nationally.

Milder diseases associated with HTLV-III/LAV infections and asymptomatic infections may be reportable in some states and cities but will not be nationally reportable. Because persons with less specific or milder manifestation of HTLV-III/LAV infection may be important in transmitting the virus, estimates of the number of such persons are of value. These estimates can be obtained through epidemiologic studies or special surveys in specific populations.

Issues related to the case definition of AIDS were discussed by the Conference of State and Territorial Epidemiologists (CSTE) at its annual meeting in Madison, Wisconsin, June 2-5, 1985. The CSTE approved the following resolutions:

1. That the case definition of AIDS used for national reporting continue to include only the more severe manifestations of HTLV-III/LAV infection; and
2. That CDC develop more inclusive definitions and classifications of HTLV-III/LAV infection for diagnosis, treatment, and prevention, as well as for epidemiologic studies and special surveys; and
3. That the following refinements be adopted in the case definition of AIDS used for national reporting:

   a. In the absence of the opportunistic diseases required by the current case definition, any of thc following diseases will be considered indicative of AIDS if the patient has a positive serologic or virologic test for HTLV-III/LAV:

      (1) disseminated histoplasmosis (not confined to lungs or lymph nodes), diagnosed by culture, histology, or antigen detection;
      (2) isosporiasis, causing chronic diarrhea (over one month), diagnosed by histology or stool microscopy;
      (3) bronchial or pulmonary candidiasis, diagnosed by microscopy or by presence of characteristic white

plaques grossly on the bronchial mucosa (not by culture alone);

(4) non-Hodgkin's lymphoma of high-grade pathologic type (diffuse, undifferentiated) and of B-cell or unknown immunologic phenotype, diagnosed by biopsy;

(5) histologically confirmed Kaposi's sarcoma in patients who are 60 years old or older when diagnosed.

b. In the absence of the opportunistic diseases required by the current case definition, a histologically confirmed diagnosis of chronic lymphoid interstitial pneumonitis in a child (under 13 years of age) will be considered indicative of AIDS unless test(s) for HTLV-III/LAV are negative.

c. Patients who have a lymphoreticular malignancy diagnosed more than three months after the diagnosis of an opportunistic disease used as a marker for AIDS will no longer be excluded as AIDS cases.

d. To increase the specificity of the case definition, patients will be excluded as AIDS cases if they have a negative result on testing for serum antibody to HTLV-III/LAV, have no other type of HTLV-III/LAV test with a positive result, and do not have a low number of T-helper lymphocytes or a low ratio of T-helper to T-suppressor lymphocytes. In the absence of test results, patients satisfying all other criteria in the definition will continue to be included.

Reported by Conference of State
and Territorial Epidemiologists;
AIDS Br, Div of Viral Diseases,
Center for Infectious Diseases, CDC

PART IV: INITIAL CDC CASE DEFINITION OF AIDS

A case definition of AIDS for national reporting was first published in 1982 by the CDC. This initial definition appeared in two articles in the *MMWR* (see Appendix A, Parts IV.A. and IV.B. below).

IV.A. Update on Acquired Immune Deficiency Syndrome (AIDS)–United States[12]

Between June 1, 1981, and September 15, 1982, CDC received reports of 593 cases of acquired immune deficiency syndrome (AIDS). Death occurred in 243 cases (41 percent).

Analysis of reported AIDS cases show that 51 percent had *Pneumocystis carinii* pneumonia (PCP) without Kaposi's sarcoma (KS) (without other "opportunistic" infections [OOI] predictive of cellular immunodeficiency); 30 percent had KS without PCP (with or without OOI); 7 percent had both PCP and KS (with or without OOI); and 12 percent had OOI with neither PCP nor KS. The overall mortality rate for cases of PCP without KS (47 percent) was more than twice that for cases of KS without PCP (21 percent), while the rate of cases of both PCP and KS (68 percent) was more than three times as great. The mortality rate for OOI with neither KS nor PCP was 48 percent.

The incidence of AIDS by date of diagnosis (assuming an almost constant population at risk) has roughly doubled every half-year since the second half of 1979. An average of one to two cases are now diagnosed every day. Although the overall case-mortality rate for the current total of 593 is 41 percent, the rate exceeds 60 percent for cases diagnosed over a year ago.

Almost 80 percent of reported AIDS cases in the United States were concentrated in six metropolitan areas, predominantly on the east and west coasts of the country. This distribution was not simply a reflection of population size in those areas; for example, the number of cases per million population reported from June 1, 1981, to September 15, 1982, in New York City and San Francisco was roughly ten times greater than that of the entire country. The 593 cases were reported among residents of 27 states and the District of Columbia, and CDC has received additional reports of 41 cases from ten foreign countries.

Approximately 75 percent of AIDS cases occurred among homosexual or bisexual males, among whom the reported prevalence of intravenous drug abuse was 12 percent. Among the 20 percent of known heterosexual cases (males and females), the prevalence of intravenous drug abuse was about 60 percent. Haitians residing in the United States constituted 6.1 percent of all cases,[13] and 50 percent of the cases in which both homosexual activity and intravenous drug abuse were denied. Among the 14 AIDS cases involving males under 60 years old who were not homosexuals, intravenous drug abusers, or Haitians, two (14 percent) had hemophilia A.[14]

Reported AIDS cases may be separated into groups based on these risk factors: homosexual or bisexual males, 75 percent; intravenous drug abusers with no history of male homosexual activity, 13 percent; Haitians with neither a history of homosexuality nor a history of intravenous drug abuse, 6 percent; persons with hemophilia A who were not Haitians, homosexual, or intravenous drug abusers, 0.3 percent; and persons in none of the other groups, 5 percent.

Reported by the Task Force
on Acquired Immune Deficiency
Syndrome, CDC

Editorial Note: CDC defines a case of AIDS as a disease, at least moderately predictive of a defect in cell-medicated immunity, occurring in a person with no known cause for diminished resistance to that disease. Such diseases include KS, PCP, and serious OOI. (These infections include pneumonia, meningitis, or encephalitis due to one or more of the following: aspergillosis, candidiasis, cryptococcosis, cytomegalovirus, nocardiosis, strongyloidosis, toxoplasmosis, zygomycosis, or atypical mycobacteriosis [species other than tuberculosis or lepra]; esophagitis due to candidiasis, cytomegalovirus, or herpes simplex virus; progressive multifocal leukoencephalopathy; chronic enterocolitis [more than four weeks] due to cryptosporidiosis; or unusually extensive mucocutaneous herpes simplex of more than five weeks duration.) Diagnoses are considered to fit the case definition only if based on sufficiently reliable methods (generally histology or culture). However, this case definition may not include the full spectrum of AIDS manifestations, which may range from absence of symptoms (despite laboratory evidence of immune deficiency) to nonspecific symptoms (e.g., fever, weight loss, generalized, persistent lymphadenopathy)[15] to specific diseases that are insufficiently predictive of cellular immunodeficiency to be included in incidence monitoring (e.g., tuberculosis, oral candidiasis, herpes zoster) to malignant neoplasms that cause, as well as result from, immunodeficiency.[16] Conversely, some patients who are considered AIDS cases on the basis of diseases only moderately predictive of cellular immunodeficiency may not actually be immunodeficient and may not be part of the current epidemic. Absence of a reliable, inexpensive, widely available test for AIDS, however, may make the working case definition the best currently available for incidence monitoring.

Two points in this update deserve emphasis. First, the eventual case-mortality rate of AIDS, a few years after diagnosis, may be far greater than the 41 percent overall case-mortality rate noted above. Second, the reported incidence of AIDS has continued to increase rapidly. Only a small percentage of cases have none of the identified risk factors (male homosexuality, intravenous drug abuse, Haitian origin, and perhaps hemophilia A). To avoid a reporting bias, physicians should report cases regardless of the absence of these factors.

IV.B. Hepatitis B Virus Vaccine Safety: Report of an Inter-Agency Group[17]

On June 25, 1982, the (ACIP) recommended using inactivated hepatitis B virus (HBV) vaccine for individuals who are at high risk for HBV infection because of their geographic origins, life styles, or exposures to HBV at home or work.[18] The recommendations included statements on vaccine efficacy and safety. However, requests for additional information on safety continue to be received, primarily because of the plasma origins of the antigen used to prepare the vaccine. In response to these requests, the Inter-Agency Group to Monitor Vaccine Development, Production and Usage, with representatives from the Centers for Disease Control (CDC), Food and Drug Administration (FDA), and National Institutes of Health (NIH), has further reviewed the available data. Its conclusions on vaccine production and safety evaluation follow.

HBV vaccine licensed in the United States is prepared from human plasma containing hepatitis surface antigen (HBsAg).[20] Hypothetical side effects from the vaccine include reactions to blood substances or to infectious agents present in donor plasma. In trials involving approximately 1,900 persons, reactions among vaccine recipients were compared with reactions among placebo recipients, and only minor immediate complaints, primarily of soreness at the injecting site, were observed.[21,22] Infectious agents that might be present in donor plasma are most likely to be viruses. Virus transmission by blood or blood products requires the virus to circulate in plasma or in cellular elements such as leukocytes. The chance of virus transmission increases with the duration of the viremic state. HBV is the only well-characterized extra-cellular human virus with a prolonged carrier state. Other agents, presumably viruses, which remain unidentified despite their common association with post-transfusion hepatitis, are responsible for non-A/non-B hepatitis.

Beginning in 1978, a disease or group of diseases was recognized, manifested by Kaposi's sarcoma and opportunist infections, associated with a specific defect in cell-mediated immunity. This group of clinical entities, along with its specific immune deficiency, is now called acquired immune deficiency syndrome (AIDS). The epidemiology of AIDS suggests an unidentified and uncharacterized blood-borne agent as a possible cause of the underlying immunologic defect.[22-24] Because AIDS occurs among populations that are sources of HBV-positive plasma, this syndrome should be considered in regard to the inherent safety of HBV vaccine.

Vaccine plasma donors are screened, and only healthy individuals (HBsAg positive) are selected. The plasmapheresis centers are licensed and inspected by the FDA. A physician gives each donor a complete physical examination, which includes a history and suitable laboratory tests. At the time of each donation, the donor's hemoglobin, hematocrit, and serum protein levels must be within normal limits. HBsAg-positive donors' levels of serum aminotransferase activity are permitted to exceed those limits set for otherwise healthy donors, but they must be stable.

The process for producing each lot of licensed HBV vaccine is designed to remove or inactivate infectious HBV and other viruses from the desired immunogen, the 22 nm HBsAg particle. The process relies on both biophysical elimination of infectious particles and treatments which inactivate viruses (pepsin at pH 2, 8M urea, and formalin). The elimination of infectious virus by biophysical purification depends on the density and flotational property of HBsAg in contrast with those of infectious virus particles. The double ultracentrifugation process (isopyknic and rate zonal) has been proven effective in removing 10^4 infectious doses of HBV/ml, as measured by chimpanzee inoculation.[25] Pepsin treatment along inactivates 10^5 or more infectious doses of HBV/ml, as measured by chimpanzee inoculation, and has been shown to inactivate viruses in the rhabdovirus, poxvirus, togavirus, reovirus, herpesvirus, and coronavirus groups.[26,27] Urea treatment alone inactivates 10^5 or more infectious doses of HBV/ml and has been shown to inactivate viruses in the rhabdovirus, myxovirus, poxvirus, togavirus, reovirus, picornavirus, herpesvirus, and coronavirus groups.[28] Slow viruses, characterized by the viruses of kuru and Creutzfeld-Jakob disease, are inactivated by 6M urea, a lesser concentration than that routinely applied to the HBV vaccine.[29] Formalin alone inactivates HBV,[30] as well as many other virus groups,[31] including parvoviruses,[32,33] retroviruses, and the delta agent.[34]

Each lot of HBV vaccine is tested for sterility, innocuousness in animals, and pyrogenicity and is free of detectable viruses, as shown by inoculation into both human and monkey cell-culture systems. Additionally, 22 doses of each vaccine lot are inoculated intravenously into four chimpanzees.

United States licensed vaccine (produced by Merck, Sharp, and Dohme) has been given to over 19,000 persons, 6,000 of whom received vaccine between October 1975 and December 1981, and 13,000 of whom received it in 1982. The vaccine has been demonstrated to protect recipients from HBV infection,[35,36] and no evidence of hepatitis has been observed as a result of HBV vaccination. Also, studies by CDC, FDA, and others of aminotransferase levels in chimpanzees and humans confirm that HBV vaccine does not transmit the non-A/non-B agents(s).

In three vaccine-placebo trials (two among homosexual men between 1978 and 1980[37,38] and one among hospital employees in 1981), 549, 714, and 664 persons, respectively, received vaccine, and equal numbers received placebo. Follow-up surveillance of participants in these studies was 24, 15, and 18 months, respectively, after the first dose of vaccine with no cases of AIDS being reported. In addition to the vaccine/placebo trials, 17,602 persons (including 8,941 health-care workers and 5,985 healthy adults, children, and infants from non-high risk group settings) have received Merck HBV vaccine in various study settings. Periods of follow-up of these vaccine recipients have ranged from a few months to over seven years. However, lots used in early studies may have been produced before the occurrence of AIDS. Some of the groups from which HBV vaccine is prepared or for which it is recommended are also at high risk for AIDS; therefore, reports of AIDS among donors and vaccinees at some future time may be expected on the basis of chance alone.

To summarize, these findings support the ACIP statement on hepatitis vaccine: (1) immediate side effects are minimal after receipt of HBV vaccine; (2) no long-term reactions have been reported; (3) the purification and inactivation process is known to inactivate representatives of all known groups of animal viruses; (4) each lot is safety tested in primates; (5) no known cases of hepatitis B or non-A/non-B hepatitis have been transmitted by the vaccine and no known occurrence of AIDS has been associated with the vaccine.

Reported by the Inter-Agency Group to Monitor Vaccine Development, Production, and Usage, represented by the Centers for Disease Control, Food and Drug Administration, and National Institutes of Health

REFERENCES

1. 1993 revised classification system for HIV infection and expanded surveillance case definition for AIDS among adolescents and adults. *MMWR–Morbidity & Mortality Weekly Report*. 41(RR-17):1-19, 1992 Dec 18.

2. CDC. Revision of the CDC surveillance case definition for acquired immunodeficiency syndrome. Council of State and Territorial Epidemiologists; AIDS Program, Center for Infectious Diseases. *MMWR–Morbidity & Mortality Weekly Report*. 36(Suppl 1):1S-15S, 1987 Aug 14.

3. CDC. Revision of the case definition of acquired immunodeficiency syndrome for national reporting–United States. *MMWR–Morbidity & Mortality Weekly Report*. 34(25):373-375, 1985 Jun 28.

4. CDC. *Pneumocystis* pneumonia–Los Angeles. *MMWR–Morbidity & Mortality Weekly Report*. 30:250-252, 1981.

5. CDC. Kaposi's sarcoma and *Pneumocystis* pneumonia among homosexual men–New York City and California. *MMWR–Morbidity & Mortality Weekly Report*. 30:305-308, 1981.

6. CDC. Hepatitis B virus vaccine safety: Report of an inter-agency group. *MMWR–Morbidity & Mortality Weekly Report*. 31:465-467, 1982.

7. CDC. Update on acquired immune deficiency syndrome (AIDS)–United States. *MMWR–Morbidity & Mortality Weekly Report*. 31:507-514, 1982.

8. Jaffe HW, Bregman DJ, Selik RM. Acquired immune deficiency syndrome in the United States: The first 1,000 cases. *Journal of Infectious Diseases*. 148:339-345, 1983.

9. Jaffe HW, Selik RM. Acquired immune deficiency syndrome: Is disseminated aspergillosis predictive of underlying cellular immune deficiency? [Reply to letter]. *Journal of Infectious Diseases*. 149:829, 1984.

10. Selik RM, Haverkos HW, Curran JW. Acquired immune deficiency syndrome (AIDS) trends in the United States, 1978-1982. *American Journal of Medicine*. 76:493-500, 1984.

11. CDC. Update: Acquired immunodeficiency syndrome (AIDS)–United States. *MMWR–Morbidity & Mortality Weekly Report*. 32:688-691, 1984.

12. CDC. Update on acquired immune deficiency syndrome (AIDS)–United States. *MMWR–Morbidity & Mortality Weekly Report*. 31(37):507-508,513-514, 1982 Sep 24.

13. CDC. Opportunistic infections and Kaposi's sarcoma among Haitians in the United States. *MMWR–Morbidity & Mortality Weekly Report*. 31:353-354, 360-361, 1982.

14. CDC. *Pneumocystis carinii* pneumonia among persons with hemophilia A. *MMWR–Morbidity & Mortality Weekly Report*. 31:365-367, 1982.

15. CDC. Persistent, generalized hymphadenophathy among homosexual males. *MMWR–Morbidity & Mortality Weekly Report*. 31:249-251, 1982.

16. CDC. Diffuse, undifferentiated non-Hodgkins hymphoma among homosexual males–United States. *MMWR–Morbidity & Mortality Weekly Report*. 31:277-279, 1982.

17. CDC. Hepatitis B virus vaccine safety: Report of an inter-agency group. *MMWR–Morbidity & Mortality Weekly Report*. 31(34):465-467, 1982 Sep 3.

18. ACIP. Inactivated hepatitis B virus vaccine. *MMWR–Morbidity & Mortality Weekly Report*. 31:317-322, 327-328, 1982.

19. Hilleman MR, Buynak EB, McAleer WJ, McLean AA, Provost PJ, Tytell A. Hepatitis A and hepatitis B vaccines, in, *Viral Hepatitis, 1981 International Symposium*, W Szmuness, HJ Alter, JE Maynard, (eds.). Philadelphia: Franklin Institute Press, 1982:385-397.

20. Szmuness W, Stevens DE, Harley EJ, Zang EA, Oleszko WR, William DC, Sadovsky R, Morrison JM, Kellner A. Hepatitis B. vaccine: Demonstration of efficacy in a controlled clinical trial in a high-risk population in the United States. *New England Journal of Medicine*. 303:833-841, 1980.

21. Francis DP, Hadler SC, Thompson SE, Maynard JE, Ostrow DG, Altman N, Braff EH, O'Malley P, Hawkins D, Judson FN, et al. The prevention of hepatitis B. with vaccine: Report of the CDC multi-center efficacy trial among homosexual men. *Annals of Internal Medicine*. 97(3):362-366, 1982 Sep.

22. CDC Task Force on Kaposi's Sarcoma and Opportunisitic Infections. Epidemiologic aspects of the current outbreak of Kaposi's sarcoma and opportunistic infections. *New England Journal of Medicine*. 306:248-252, 1982.

23. CDC. *Pneumocystis carinii* pneumonia among persons with hemophilia A. *MMWR–Morbidity & Mortality Weekly Report*. 31:365-367, 1982.

24. Fauci AS. The syndrome of Kaposi's sarcoma and opportunistic infections: An epidemiologically restricted disorder of immunoregulation. *Annals of Internal Medicine*. 96:777-779, 1982.

25. Gerety RJ, Tabor E, Purcell RH, Tyeryar FJ. Summary of an international workshop on hepatitis B vaccines. *Journal of Infectious Diseases*. 140:642-648, 1979.

26. Tabor E, Buynak E, Smallwood LA, Suoy P, Hilleman M, Gerety RJ. Inactivation of hepatitis B virus by three methods: Treatment with pepsin, urea, or formalin. *Journal of Medical Virology*. 11(1):1-9, 1983.

27. Buynak EB, Roehm RR, Tytell AA, Bertland AU, Lampson GP, Hilleman MR. Development and chimpanzee testing of a vaccine against human hepatitis B. *Proceedings of the Society for Experimental Biology and Medicine*. 151:694-700, 1976.

28. Tabor E, Buynak E, Smallwood LA, Suoy P, Hilleman M, Gerety RJ. Inactivation of hepatitis B virus by three methods: Treatment with pepsin, urea, or formalin. *Journal of Medical Virology*. 11(1):1-9, 1983.

29. Gajdusek DC. Unconventional viruses and the origin and disappearance of kuru. *Science*. 197:943-960, 1977.

30. Tabor E, Buynak E, Smallwood LA, Suoy P, Hilleman M, Gerety RJ. Inactivation of hepatitis B virus by three methods: Treatment with pepsin, urea, or formalin. *Journal of Medical Virology*. 11(1):1-9, 1983.

31. Eugster AK. Studies on canine parvovirus infections: Development of an inactivated vaccine. *American Journal of Veterinary Research*. 41:2020-2024, 1980.

32. Gross L. *Oncogenic viruses*. New York: Pergamon Press, 1961.

33. Walker JF. *Formaldehyde*. 3rd ed. Huntington, NY: Krieger, 1975:395-404, 601-603.

34. Purcell, R. Unpublished data.

35. Szmuness W, Stevens CE, Harley EJ, Zang EA, Oleszko WR, William DC, Sadovsky R, Morrison JM, Kellner A. Hepatitis B vaccine: Demonstration of efficacy in a controlled clinical trial in a high-risk population in the United States. *New England Journal of Medicine*. 303:833-841, 1980.

36. Francis DP, Hadler SC, Thompson SE, Maynard JE, Ostrow DG, Altman N, Braff EH, O'Malley P, Hawkins D, Judson FN, et al. The prevention of hepatitis B with vaccine: Report of the CDC multi-center efficacy trial among homosexual men. *Annals of Internal Medicine*. 97(3):362-366, Sep 1982.

37. Szmuness W, Stevens CE, Harley EJ, Zang EA, Oleszko WA, William DC, Sadosky R, Morrison JM, Kellner A. Hepatitis B vaccine: Demonstration of efficacy in a controlled clinical trial in a high-risk population in the United States. *New England Journal of Medicine*. 303:833-841, 1980.

38. Francis DP, Hadler SC, Thompson SE, Maynard JE, Ostrow DG, Altman N, Braff EH, O'Malley P, Hawkins D, Judson FN, et al. The prevention of hepatitis B with vaccine: Report of the CDC multi-center efficacy trial among homosexual men. *Annals of Internal Medicine*. 97(3):362-366, Sep 1982.

Appendix B

AIDS Classification Systems

This appendix contains the selective text of the CDC and the Walter Reed AIDS classification systems as they appeared in the published literature (see the original articles for the complete text). While other classification systems have been proposed, these two remain the most widely accepted. The CDC classification system was published first in 1986, and has been revised to reflect a better understanding of the manifestations of HIV and AIDS.

PART I:
1993 CDC REVISED HIV CLASSIFICATION SYSTEM FOR ADOLESCENTS AND ADULTS[1]

The etiologic agent of acquired immunodeficiency syndrome (AIDS) is a retrovirus designated human immunodeficiency virus (HIV). The CD4+ T-lymphocyte is the primary target for HIV infection because of the affinity of the virus for the CD4 surface marker.[2] The CD4+ T-lymphocyte coordinates a number of important immunologic functions, and a loss of these functions results in progressive impairment of the immune response. Studies of the natural history of HIV infection have documented a wide spectrum of disease manifestations, ranging from asymptomatic infection to life-threatening conditions characterized by severe immunodeficiency, serious opportunistic infections, and cancers.[3-12] Other studies have shown a strong association between the development of life-threatening opportunistic illnesses and the absolute number (per microliter of blood) or percentage of CD4+ T-lymphocytes.[13-20] As the number of CD4+ T-lymphocytes decreases, the risk and severity of opportunistic illnesses increase.

Measures of CD4+ T-lymphocytes are used to guide clinical and therapeutic management of HIV-infected persons.[21] Antimicrobial prophylaxis and antiretroviral therapies have been shown to be most effective within certain levels of immune dysfunction.[22-27] As a result, antiretroviral therapy should be considered for all persons with CD4+ T-lymphocyte counts of <500/cubic millimeter, and prophylaxis against *Pneumocystis carinii* pneumonia (PCP), the most common serious opportunistic infection diagnosed in men and women with AIDS, is recommended for all persons with CD4+ T-lymphocyte counts of <200/cubic millimeter and for persons who have had prior episodes of PCP. Because of these recommendations, CD4+ T-lymphocyte determinations are an integral part of medical management of HIV-infected persons in the United States.

The classification system for HIV infection among adolescents and adults has been revised to include the CD4+ T-lymphocyte count as a marker for HIV-related immunosuppression. This revision establishes mutually exclusive subgroups for which the spectrum of clinical conditions is integrated with the CD4+ T-lymphocyte count. The objectives of these changes are to simplify the classification of HIV infection, to reflect current standards of medical care for HIV-infected persons, and to categorize more accurately HIV-related morbidity.

The revised CDC classification system for HIV-infected adolescents and adults* categorizes persons on the basis of clinical

---

***Criteria for HIV infection for persons age ≥13 years:** (a) repeatedly reactive screening tests for HIV antibody (e.g., enzyme immunoassay) with specific antibody identified by the use of supplemental tests (e.g., Western blot, immunofluorescence assay); (b) direct identification of virus in host tissues by virus isolation; (c) HIV antigen detection; or (d) a positive result on any other highly specific licensed test for HIV.

conditions associated with HIV infection and CD4+ T-lymphocyte counts. The system is based on three ranges of CD4+ T-lymphocyte counts and three clinical categories and is represented by a matrix of nine mutually exclusive categories. This system replaces the classification system published in 1986, which included only clinical disease criteria and which was developed before the widespread use of CD4+ T-cell testing.[28]

CD4+ T-Lymphocyte Categories

The three CD4+ T-lymphocyte categories are defined as follows:

- **Category 1:** ≥500 cells/cubic millimeter
- **Category 2:** 200-499 cells/cubic millimeter
- **Category 3:** <200 cells/cubic millimeter

These categories correspond to CD4+ T-lymphocyte counts per microliter of blood, and guide clinical and therapeutic ac-tions in the management of HIV-infected adolescents and adults.[29-35] The revised HIV classification system also allows for the use of the percentage of CD4+ T-cells (see Appendix A, Part I.A.).

HIV-infected persons should be classified based on existing guidelines for the medical management of HIV-infected persons.[36] Thus, the lowest accurate, but not necessarily the most recent, CD4+T-lymphocyte count should be used for classification purposes.

Clinical Categories

The clinical categories of HIV infection are defined as follows:

Category A

Category A consists of one or more of the conditions listed below in adolescents or adult (>13 years) with documented HIV infection. Conditions listed in Categories B and C must not have occurred.

- Asymptomatic HIV infection
- Persistent generalized lymphadenopathy
- Acute (primary) HIV infection with accompanying illness or history of acute HIV infection

Category B

Category B consists of symptomatic conditions in an HIV-infected adolescent or adult that are not included among conditions listed in clinical Category C and that meet at least one of the following criteria: (a) the conditions are attributed to HIV infection or are indicative of a defect in cell-mediated immunity; or (b) the conditions are considered by physicians to have a clinical course or to require management that is complicated by HIV infection. **Examples** of conditions in clinical Category B include, **but are not limited to**:

- Bacillary angiomatosis
- Candidiasis, oropharyngeal (thrush)
- Candidiasis, vulvovaginal; persistent, frequent, or poorly responsive to therapy
- Cervical dysplasia (moderate or severe)/cervical carcinoma in situ
- Constitutional symptoms, such as fever (38.5 C) or diarrhea lasting >1 month
- Hairy leukoplakia, oral
- Herpes Zoster (shingles), involving at least two distinct episodes or more than one dermatome
- Idiopathic thrombocytopenic purpura
- Listeriosis
- Pelvic inflammatory disease, particularly if complicated by tubo-ovarian abscess
- Peripheral neuropathy

For classification purposes, Category B conditions take precedence over those in Category A. For example, someone previously treated for oral or persistent vaginal candidiasis (and who has not developed a Category C disease) but who is now asymptomatic should be classified in clinical Category B.

Category C

Category C includes the clinical conditions listed in the AIDS surveillance case definition (see Appendix A, Part I.B.). For classification purposes, once a Category C condition has occurred, the person will remain in Category C.

PART II: CLASSIFICATION SYSTEM FOR HUMAN IMMUNODEFICIENCY VIRUS (HIV) INFECTION IN CHILDREN UNDER 13 YEARS OF AGE[37]

Introduction

With the identification of the causative agent of the acquired immunodeficiency syndrome (AIDS), a broad spectrum of clinical manifestations has been attributed to infection with the human immunodeficiency virus (HIV). With the exception of the CDC surveillance definition for AIDS,[38,39] no standard definitions for other manifestations of HIV infection have been developed for children. Classification systems published to date have been developed primarily to categorize clinical presentations in adult patients and may not be entirely applicable to infants and children.[40-42]

Physicians from institutions caring for relatively large numbers of HIV-infected children report that only about half of their patients with symptomatic illness related to the infection fulfill the criteria of the CDC surveillance definition for AIDS.[43,44]

To develop a classification system for HIV infection in children, CDC convened a panel of consultants consisting of clinicians experienced in the diagnosis and management of children with HIV infection; public health physicians; and representatives from the American Academy of Pediatrics, the Council of State and Territorial Epidemiologists, the Association for Maternal Child Health and Crippled Children's Programs, the National Institute on Drug Abuse/Alcohol, Drug Abuse and Mental Health Administration, the National Institute of Allergy and Infectious Diseases/National Institutes of Health, and the Division of Maternal and Child Health/Health Resources and Services Administration and CDC.

Goals and Objectives of the Classification System

The system was designed primarily for public health purposes, including epidemiologic studies, disease surveillance, prevention programs, and health-care planning and policy. The panel attempted to devise a simple scheme that could be subdivided as needed for different purposes.

Definition of HIV Infection in Children (Table 2)

Ideally, HIV infection in children is identified by the presence of the virus in blood or tissues, confirmed by culture or other laboratory detection methods. However, current tests–including culture–for detecting the virus or its antigens are not standardized and are not readily available. Detection of specific antibody to the virus is a sensitive and specific indicator of HIV infection in adults, since the majority of adults with antibody have had culture evidence of infection.[45-47] Similar studies involving children have not been reported. Also, the presence of passively transferred maternal antibody in infants limits the interpretation of a positive antibody test result in this age group. Most of the consultants believed that passively transferred maternal HIV antibody could sometimes persist for up to 15 months. For this reason, two definitions for infection in children are needed: one for infants and children up to 15 months of age who have been exposed to their infected mothers perinatally, and another for older children with perinatal infection and for infants and children of all ages acquiring the virus through other means.

Infants and Children under 15 Months of Age with Perinatal Infection

Infection in infants and children up to 15 months of age who were exposed to infected mothers in the perinatal period may be defined by one or more of the following: (1) the identification of the virus in blood or tissues, (2) the presence of HIV antibody as indicated by a repeatedly reactive screening test (e.g., enzyme immunoassay) plus a positive confirmatory test (e.g., Western blot, immunofluorescence assay) in an infant or child who has abnormal immunologic test results indicating both humoral and cellular immunodeficiency (increased immunoglobulin levels, depressed T4 [T-helper] absolute cell count, absolute lymphopenia, decreased T4/T8 ratio) and who meets the requirements of one or more of the subclasses listed under class P-2 (described below), or (3) the confirmation that a child's symptoms meet the previously published CDC case definition for pediatric AIDS.[48,49]

The infection status of other perinatally exposed seropositive infants and children up to 15 months of age who lack one of the above immunologic or clinical criteria is indeterminate. These infants should be followed up for HIV-related illness, and they should be tested at regular intervals for persistence of antibody to HIV. Infants and children who become seronegative, are virus-culture negative (if blood or tissue samples are cultured), and continue to have no clinical or laboratory-confirmed abnormalities associated with HIV infection are unlikely to be infected.

Older Children with Perinatal Infection and Children with HIV Infection Acquired Through Other Modes of Transmission

HIV infection in these children is defined by one or more of the following: (1) the identification of virus in blood or tissues; (2) the presence of HIV antibody (positive screening test plus confirmatory test) regardless of whether immunologic abnormalities or signs or symptoms are present; or (3) the confirmation that the child's symptoms meet the previously published CDC case definition for Pediatric AIDS.[50,51]

These definitions apply to children under 13 years of age. Persons 13 years of age and older should be classified according to the adult classification system.[52]

Table 2. Summary of the Definition of HIV Infection in Children

Infants and children under 15 months of age with perinatal infection

1. Virus in blood or tissues
   or
2. HIV antibody
   and
   evidence of both cellular and humoral immune deficiency
   and
   one or more categories in Class P-2
   or
3. Symptoms meeting CDC case definition for AIDS

Older Children with perinatal infection and children with HIV infection acquired through other modes of transmission

1. Virus in blood or tissues
   or
2. HIV antibody
   or
3. Symptoms meeting CDC case definition for AIDS

Classification System (Table 3)

Children fulfilling the definition of HIV infection discussed above may be classified into one of two mutually exclusive classes based on the presence or absence of clinical signs and symptoms (Table 3). Class Pediatric-1 (P-1) is further subcategorized on the basis of the presence or absence of immunologic abnormalities, whereas Class P-2 is subdivided by specific disease patterns. Once a child has signs and symptoms and is therefore classified in P-2, he or she should not be reassigned to class P-1 if signs and symptoms resolve.

Perinatally exposed infants and children whose infection status is indeterminate are classified into class P-0.

Class P-0: Indeterminate Infection

Includes perinatally exposed infants and children up to 15 months of age who cannot be classified as definitely infected according to the above definition but who have antibody to HIV, indicating exposure to a mother who is infected.

Class P-1: Asymptomatic Infection

Includes patients who meet one of the above definitions for HIV infection but who have had no previous signs or symptoms that would have led to classification in Class P-2.

These children may be subclassified on the basis of immunologic testing. This testing should include quantitative immunoglobulins, complete blood count with differential, and T-lymphocyte subset quantitation. Results of functional testing of lymphocytes (mitogens, such as pokeweed) may also be abnormal in HIV-infected children, but it is less specific in comparison with immunoglobulin levels and lymphocyte subset analysis, and it may be impractical.

Subclass A–Normal immune function. Includes children with no immune abnormalities associated with HIV infection.

Subclass B–Abnormal immune function. Includes children with one or more of the commonly observed immune abnormalities associated with HIV infection, such as hypergammaglobulinemia, T-helper (T4) lymphopenia, decreased T-helper/T-suppressor (T4/T8) ratio, and absolute lymphopenia. Other causes of these abnormalities must be excluded.

Subclass C–Not tested. Includes children for whom no or incomplete (see above) immunologic testing has been done.

Class P-2: Symptomatic Infection

Includes patients meeting the above definitions for HIV infection and having signs and symptoms of infection. Other causes of these signs and symptoms should be excluded. Subclasses are defined based on the type of signs and symptoms that are present. Patients may be classified in more than one subclass.

Subclass A–Nonspecific findings. Includes children with two or more unexplained nonspecific findings persisting for more than two months, including fever, failure-to-thrive or weight loss of more than 10 percent of baseline, hepatomegaly, splenomegaly, generalized lymphadenopathy (lymph nodes measuring at least 0.5 cm present in two or more sites, with bilateral lymph nodes counting as one site), parotitis, and diarrhea (three or more loose stools per day) that is either persistent or recurrent (defined as two or more episodes of diarrhea accompanied by dehydration within a two-month period).

Subclass B–Progressive neurologic disease. Includes children with one or more of the following progressive findings: (1) loss of developmental milestones or intellectual ability; (2) impaired brain growth (acquired microcephaly and/or brain atrophy demonstrated on computerized tomographic scan or magnetic resonance imaging scan); or (3) progressive symmetrical motor deficits manifested by two or more of these findings: paresis, abnormal tone, pathologic reflexes, ataxia, or gait disturbance.

Subclass C–Lymphoid interstitial pneumonitis. Includes children with a histologically confirmed pneumonitis characterized by diffuse interstitial and peribronchiolar infiltration of lymphocytes and plasma cells and without identifiable pathogens, or, in the absence of a histologic diagnosis, a chronic pneumonitis–characterized by bilateral reticulonodular interstitial infiltrates with or without hilar lymphadenopathy–present on chest x-ray for a period of at least two months and unresponsive to appropriate antimicrobial therapy. Other causes of interstitial infiltrates should be excluded, such as tuberculosis, *Pneumocystis carinii* pneumonia, cytomegalovirus infection, or other viral or parasitic infections.

Subclass D–Secondary infectious diseases. Includes children with a diagnosis of an infectious disease that occurs as a result of immune deficiency caused by infection with HIV.

Category D-1. Includes patients with secondary infectious disease due to one of the specified infectious diseases listed in the CDC surveillance definition for AIDS: *Pneumocystis carinii* pneumonia; chronic cryptosporidiosis; disseminated toxoplasmosis with onset after one month of age; extra-intestinal strongyloidiasis; chronic isosporiasis; candidiasis (esophageal bronchial, or pulmonary); extrapulmonary cryptococcosis; disseminated histoplasmosis; noncutaneous, extrapulmonary, or disseminated mycobacterial infection (any species other than leprae); cytomegalovirus infection with onset after one month of age; chronic mucocutaneous or disseminated herpes simplex virus infection with onset after one month of age; extrapulmonary or disseminated coccidioidomycosis; nocardiosis; and progressive multifocal leukoencephalopathy.

Category D-2. Includes patients with unexplained, recurrent, serious arterial infections (two or more within a two-year period) including sepsis, meningitis, pneumonia, abscess of an internal organ, and bone/joint infections.

Category D-3. Includes patients with other infectious disease, including oral candidiasis persisting for two months or more, two or more episodes of herpes stomatitis within a year, or multidermatomal or disseminated herpes zoster infection.

Subclass E–Secondary cancers. Includes children with any cancer described below in Categories E-1 and E-2.

Category E-1. Includes patients with the diagnosis of one or more kinds of cancer known to be associated with HIV infection as listed in the surveillance definition of AIDS and indicative of a defect in cell-mediated immunity: Kaposi's sarcoma, B-cell non-Hodgkin's lymphoma, or primary lymphoma of the brain.

Category E-2. Includes patients with the diagnosis of other malignancies possibly associated with HIV infection.

Subclass F–Other diseases. Includes children with other conditions possibly due to HIV infection not listed in the above subclasses, such as hepatitis, cardiopathy, nephropathy, hematologic disorders (anemia, thrombocytopenia), and dermatologic diseases.

Table 3. Summary of the Classification of HIV Infection in Children under 13 Years of Age

Class P-0: Indeterminate infection

Class P-1: Asymptomatic infection

Subclass A. Normal immune function
Subclass B. Abnormal immune function
Subclass C. Immune function not tested

Class P-2: Symptomatic infection

Subclass A. Nonspecific findings

Subclass B. Progressive neurologic disease
Subclass C. Lymphoid interstitial pneumonitis
Subclass D. Secondary infectious diseases
- Category D-1 Specified secondary infectious diseases listed in the CDC surveillance definition for AIDS
- Category D-2 Recurrent serious bacterial infections
- Category D-3 Other specified secondary infectious diseases

Subclass E. Secondary cancers
- Category E-1. Specified secondary cancers listed in the CDC surveillance definition for AIDS
- Category E-2. Other cancers possibly secondary to HIV infection

Subclass F. Other diseases possibly due to HIV infection

Reported by AIDS Program,
Center for Infectious Diseases, CDC

Editorial Note: This classification system is based on present knowledge and understanding of pediatric HIV infection and may need to be revised as new information becomes available. New diagnostic tests, particularly antigen detection tests and HIV-specific IgM tests, may lead to a better definition of HIV infection in infants and children. Information from several natural history studies currently under way may necessitate changes in the subclasses based on clinical signs and symptoms.

A definitive diagnosis of HIV infection in perinatally exposed infants and children under 15 months of age can be difficult. The infection status of these HIV-seropositive infants and children who are asymptomatic without immune abnormalities cannot be determined unless virus culture or other antigen-detection tests are positive. Negative virus cultures do not necessarily mean the child is not infected, since the sensitivity of the culture may be low. Decreasing antibody titers have been helpful in diagnosing other perinatal infections, such as toxoplasmosis and cytomegalovirus. However, the pattern of HIV-antibody production in infants is not well defined. At present, close follow-up of these children (Class P-0) for signs and symptoms indicative of HIV infection and/or persistence of HIV antibody is recommended.

The parents of children with HIV infection should be evaluated for HIV infection, particularly the mother. The child is often the first person in such families to become symptomatic. When HIV infection in a chid is suspected, a careful history should be taken to elicit possible risk factors for the parents and the child. Appropriate laboratory tests, including HIV serology, should be offered. If the mother is seropositive, other children should be evaluated regarding their risk of perinatally acquired infection. Intrafamilial transmission, other than perinatal or sexual, is extremely unlikely. Identification of other infected family members allows for appropriate medical care and prevention of transmission to sexual partners and future children.[53,54]

PART III: CLASSIFICATION SYSTEM FOR HUMAN T-LYMPHOTROPIC VIRUS TYPE III/LYMPHADENOPATHY-ASSOCIATED VIRUS INFECTIONS[55]

Introduction

Persons infected with the etiologic retrovirus of acquired immunodeficiency syndrome (AIDS)[56-59] may present with a variety of manifestations ranging from asymptomatic infection to severe immunodeficiency and life-threatening secondary infectious diseases or cancers. The rapid growth of knowledge about human T-lymphotropic virus type III/lymphadenopathy-associated virus (HTLV-III/LAV) has resulted in an increasing need for a system of classifying patients within this spectrum of clinical and laboratory findings attributable to HTLV-III/LAV infection.[60-62]

Various means are now used to describe and assess patients with manifestations of HTLV-III/LAV infection and to describe their signs, symptoms, and laboratory findings. The surveillance definitions of AIDS has proven to be extremely valuable and quite reliable for some epidemiologic studies and clinical assessment of patients with the more severe manifestations of disease. However, more inclusive definitions and classifications of HTLV-III/LAV infection are need for optimum patient care, health planning, and public health control strategies, as well as for epidemic studies and special surveys. A broadly applicable, easily understood classification system should also facilitate and clarify communication about this disease.

In an attempt to formulate the most appropriate classification system, CDC has sought the advice of a panel of expert consultants to assist in defining the manifestations of HTLV-III/LAV infection.

Goals and Objectives of the Classification System

The classification system presented in this report is primarily applicable to public health purposes, including disease reporting and surveillance, epidemiologic studies, prevention and control activities, and public health policy and planning.

Immediate applications of such a system include the classification of infected persons for reporting of cases to state and local public health agencies, and use in various disease coding and recording systems, such as the forthcoming tenth revision of the International Classification of Diseases.

Definition of HTLV-III/LAV Infection

The most specific diagnosis of HTLV-III/LAV infection is by direct identification of the virus in host tissues by virus isolation; however, the techniques for isolating HTLV-III/LAV currently lack sensitivity for detecting infection and are not readily available. For public health purposes, patients with repeatedly reactive screening tests for HTLV-III/LAV antibody (e.g., enzyme-linked immunosorbent assay) in whom antibody is also identified by the use of supplemental tests (e.g., Western blot, immunofluorescence assay) should be considered both infected and infective.[63-65]

Although HTLV-III/LAV infection is identified by isolation of the virus or, indirectly, by the presence of antibody to the virus, a presumptive clinical diagnosis of HTLV-III/LAV infection has been made in some situations in the absence of positive virologic or serologic test results. There is a very strong correlation between the clinical manifestations of AIDS as defined by CDC and the presence of HTLV-III/LAV antibody.[66-69] Most persons whose clinical illness fulfills the CDC surveillance definition for AIDS will have been infected with the virus.[70-72]

Classification System

This system classifies the manifestations of HTLV-III/LAV infection into four mutually exclusive groups, designated by Roman numerals I through IV (Table 4). *The classification system applies only to patients diagnosed as having HTLV-III/LAV infection (see previous section,* **Definition of HTLV-III/LAV Infection***).* Classification in a particular group is not explicitly intended to have prognostic significance, nor to designate severity of illness. However, classification in the four principal groups, I through IV, is hierarchical in that persons classified in a particular group should not be reclassified in a preceding group if clinical findings resolve, since clinical improvement may not accurately reflect changes in the severity of the underlying disease.

Group I includes patients with transient signs and symptoms that appear at the time of, or shortly after, initial infection with HTLV-III/LAV as identified by laboratory studies. All patients in Group I will be reclassified in another group following resolution of this acute syndrome.

Group II includes patients who have no signs or symptoms of HTLV-III/LAV infection. Patients in this category may be subclassified based on whether hematologic and/or immunologic laboratory studies have been done and whether results are abnormal in a manner consistent with the effects of HTLV-III/LAV infection.

Group III includes patients with persistent generalized lymphadenopathy, but without findings that would lead to classification in Group IV. Patients in this category may be subclassified based on the results of laboratory studies in the same manner as patients in Group II.

Group IV includes patients with clinical symptoms and signs of HTLV-III/LAV infection other than or in addition to lymphadenopathy. Patients in this group are assigned to one or more subgroups based on clinical findings. These are: Subgroup A, constitutional disease; Subgroup B, neurologic disease; Subgroup C, Secondary infectious diseases; Subgroup D, secondary cancers; and Subgroup E, other conditions resulting from HTLV-III/LAV infection. There is no a priori hierarchy of severity among subgroups A through E, and these subgroups are not mutually exclusive.

Definitions of the groups and subgroups are as follows:

Group I: Acute HTLV-III/LAV Infection

Defined as a mononucleosis-like syndrome, with or without aseptic meningitis, associated with seroconversion for HTLV-III/LAV antibody.[73,74] Antibody seroconversion is required as evidence of initial infection; current viral isolation procedures are not adequately sensitive to be relied on for demonstrating the onset of infection.

Group II: Asymptomatic HTLV-III/LAV Infection

Defined as the absence of signs or symptoms of HTLV-III/LAV infection. To be classified in Group II, patients must have had no previous signs or symptoms that would have led to classification in Groups III or IV. Patients whose clinical findings caused them to be classified in Groups III or IV should not be reclassified in Group II if those clinical findings resolve.

Patients in this group may be subclassified on the basis of a laboratory evaluation. Laboratory studies commonly indicated for patients with HTLV-III/LAV infection include, but are not limited to, a complete blood count (including differential white blood cell count) and a platelet count. Immunologic tests, especially T-lymphocyte helper and suppressor cell counts, are also an important part of the overall evaluation. Patients whose test results are within normal limits, as well as those for whom a laboratory evaluation has not yet been completed, should be differentiated from patients whose test results are consistent with defects associated with HTLV-III/LAV infection (e.g., lymphopenia, thrombocytopenia, decreased number of helper [T4] T-lymphocytes).

Group III: Persistent Generalized Lymphadenopathy (PGL)

Defined as palpable lymphadenopathy (lymph node enlargement of 1 cm or greater) at two or more extra-inguinal sites persisting for more than three months in the absence of a concurrent illness or condition other than HTLV-III/LAV infection to explain the findings. Patients in this group may also be subclassified on the basis of a laboratory evaluation, as is done for asymptomatic patients in Group II (see above). Patients with PGL whose clinical findings caused them to be classified in Group IV should not be reclassified in Group III if those other clinical findings resolve.

Group IV: Other HTLV-III/LAV Diseases

The clinical manifestations of patients in this group may be designated by assignment to one or more subgroups (A through E) listed below. Within Group IV, subgroup classification is independent of the presence or absence of lymphadenopathy. Each subgroup may include patients who are minimally symptomatic, as well as patients who are severely ill. Increased specificity for manifestations of

HTLV-III/LAV infection, if needed for clinical purposes or research purposes or for disability determinations, may be achieved by creating additional divisions within each subgroup.

Subgroup A–Constitutional disease. Defined as one or more of the following: fever persisting more than one month, involuntary weight loss of greater than 10 percent of baseline, or diarrhea persisting more than one month; and the absence of a concurrent illness or condition other than HTLV-III/LAV infection to explain the findings.

Subgroup B–Neurologic disease. Defined as one or more of the following: dementia, myelopathy, or peripheral neuropathy; and the absence of a concurrent illness or condition other than HTLV-III/LAV infection to explain the findings.

Subgroup C–Secondary infectious diseases. Defined as the diagnosis of an infectious disease associated with HTLV-III/LAV infection and/or at least moderately indicative of a defect in cell-mediated immunity. Patients in this subgroup are divided further into two categories:

> *Category C-1.* Includes patients with symptomatic or invasive disease due to one of 12 specified secondary infectious diseases listed in the surveillance definition of AIDS: *Pneumocystis carinii* pneumonia, chronic cryptosporidiosis, toxoplasmosis, extra-intestinal strongyloidiasis, isosporiasis, candidiasis (esophageal, bronchial, or pulmonary), cryptococcosis, histoplasmosis, mycobacterial infection with *Mycobacterium avium* complex or *M. kansasii,* cytomegalovirus infection, chronic mucocutaneous or disseminated herpes simplex virus infection, and progressive multifocal leukoencephalopathy.
>
> *Category C-2.* Includes patients with symptomatic or invasive disease due to one of six other specified secondary infectious diseases: oral hairy leukoplakia, multidermatomal herpes zoster, recurrent *Salmonella* bacteremia, nocardiosis, tuberculosis, or oral candidiasis (thrush).

Subgroup D–Secondary cancers. Defined as the diagnosis of one or more kinds of cancer known to be associated with HTLV-III/LAV infection as listed in the surveillance definition of AIDS and at least moderately indicative of a defect in cell-mediated immunity: Kaposi's sarcoma, non-Hodgkin's lymphoma (small, noncleaved lymphoma or immunoblastic sarcoma), or primary lymphoma of the brain.

Subgroup E–Other conditions in HTLV-III/LAV infection. Defined as the presence of other clinical findings or diseases, not classifiable above, that may be attributed to HTLV-III/LAV infection and/or may be indicative of a defect in cell-mediated immunity. Included are patients with chronic lymphoid interstitial pneumonitis. Also included are those patients whose signs or symptoms could be attributed either to HTLV-III/LAV infection or to another coexisting disease not classified elsewhere, and patients with other clinical illnesses, the course or management of which may be complicated or altered by HTLV-III/LAV infection. Examples include: patients with constitutional symptoms not meeting the criteria for Subgroup IV-A; patients with infectious diseases not listed in Subgroup IV-C; and patients with neoplasms not listed in Subgroup IV-D.

Table 4. Summary of Classification System for Human T-lymphotropic Virus Type III/Lymphadenopathy-Associated Virus

Group I. Acute infection

Group II. Asymptomatic infection*

Group III. Persistent generalized lymphadenopathy*

Group IV. Other disease

---

*Patients in Groups II and III may be subclassified on the basis of a laboratory evaluation.

Subgroup A. Constitutional disease
Subgroup B. Neurologic disease
Subgroup C. Secondary infectious diseases
  Category C-1. Specified secondary infectious diseases listed in the CDC surveillance definition for AIDS
  Category C-2. Other specified secondary infectious diseases
Subgroup D. Secondary cancers
Subgroup E. Other conditions

Reported by
Center for Infectious Diseases, CDC

Editorial Note: The classification system is meant to provide a means of grouping patients infected with HTLV-III/LAV according to the clinical expression of disease. It will require periodic revision as warranted by new information about HTLV-III/LAV infection. The definition of particular syndromes will evolve with increasing knowledge of the significance of certain clinical findings and laboratory tests. New diagnostic techniques, such as the detection of specific HTLV-III/LAV antigens or antibodies, may add specificity to the assessment of patients infected with HTLV-III/LAV.

The classification system defines a limited number of specified clinical presentations. Patients whose signs and symptoms do not meet the criteria for other groups and subgroups, but whose findings are attributable to HTLV-III/LAV infection, should be classified in Subgroup IV-E. As the classification system is revised and updated, certain subsets of patients in Subgroup IV-E may be identified as having related groups of clinical findings that should be separately classified as distinct syndromes. This could be accomplished either by creating additional subgroups within Group IV or by broadening the definitions of the existing subgroups.

Persons currently using other classification systems[75,76] or nomenclatures (e.g., AIDS-related complex, lymphadenopathy syndrome) can find equivalences with those systems and terminologies and the classification presented in this report. Because this classification system has only four principal groups based on chronology, presence or absence of signs and symptoms, and the type of clinical findings present, comparisons with other classifications based either on clinical findings or on laboratory assessment are easily accomplished.

This classification system does not imply any change in the definition of AIDS used by CDC since 1981 for national reporting. Patients whose clinical presentations fulfill the surveillance definition of AIDS are classified in Group IV. However, not every case in Group IV will meet the surveillance definition.

PART IV: THE WALTER REED STAGING CLASSIFICATION FOR HTLV-III/LAV INFECTION[77]

In 1985, the United States Army adopted a staging classification for HTLV-III/LAV infection. The staging classification system was implemented to ensure uniformity for clinical evaluations of patients, to gain a better understanding of these infections, and to help evaluate the clinical response to treatment regimens initiated against these infections. This staging scheme is only applicable to adults, as it is based on adult base-line functional T-cell indexes. This system is based on two key observations: (1) the T helper (T4) cell is the primary target of the virus; and (2) the degree to which the T helper (T4) cell is functionally impaired determines the clinical presentation of the illness. The scheme does not assume that all patients will have progressive disease.

The Walter Reed (WR) staging classification system ranges from Stage 0 to Stage 6, with WR0 showing no signs of infection with the causative agent for AIDS and WR6 indicating the presence of the causative agent for AIDS and the presence of at least one opportunistic infection (see Table 5). Stage WR0 is indicative of potential exposure through high-risk contact; Stages WR1 through WR6 require documentation of infection by demonstration of the presence of antibodies using a Western blot or comparable assay. Letters representing a particular condition or opportunistic infection are added to the appropriate stage designation to complete the stage description (e.g., WR4K represents a patient who meets the criteria for Stage 4 and has Kaposi's sarcoma). *K* is used to represent Kaposi's sarcoma; *N* is used to represent neoplasms other than Kaposi's sarcoma; *B* is used to represent constitutional symptoms such as temperature, night sweats, or weight loss; and *CNS* is used to represent neurologic manifestations.

For the purpose of the Walter Reed staging classification system, chronic lymphadenopathy is defined as the presence of two or more extraingiunal lymph node sites that are at least one centimeter in diameter persisting for a minimum of three months. A decrease in T helper (T4) cells is defined as <400/cubic millimeter persisting for a minimum of three months. Delayed hypersensitivity is defined as normal (induration of at least five millimeters) to a minimum of two of the following four antigen tests: candida, mumps, tetanus, trichophyton. Partial anergy is response to only one antigen, whereas complete anergy is a complete lack of response. Thrush is defined as clinical oral candidiasis, with a positive potassium hydroxide preparation or Gram stain showing masses of hyphae, pseudohyphae, and yeast forms denoting a positive diagnosis. Opportunistic infections include chronic mucocutaneous herpes simplex, disseminated cytomegalovirus, disseminated histoplasmosis, candida esophagitis, disseminated nocardiosis, *Pneumocystis carinii* pneumonia, central nervous system (CNS) or disseminated toxoplasmosis, chronic cryptosporidiosis, CNS or disseminated cryptococcosis, disseminated atypical mycobacterial disease, and extrapulmonary tuberculosis. Kaposi's sarcoma does not qualify as an opportunistic infection and does not qualify for WR6 classification because it can occur without severe T helper (T4) cell depletion.

Table 5. The Walter Reed Staging Classification for HTLV-III/LAV Infection

Stage	Criteria
WR0	No presence of antibodies for HTLV-III/LAV and T4 count >400
WR1	HTLV-III/LAV antibody positive test
WR2	HTLV-III/LAV antibody positive test Chronic lymphadenopathy
WR3	HTLV-III/LAV antibody positive test Chronic lymphadenopathy T4 count <400
WR4	HTLV-III/LAV antibody positive test Chronic lymphadenopathy T4 count <400 Partial anergy
WR5	HTLV-III/LAV antibody positive test Chronic lymphadenopathy T4 count <400 Partial/complete anergy +/- Thrush
WR6	HTLV-III/LAV antibody positive test Chronic lymphadenopathy T4 count <400 Partial/complete anergy +/- Thrush Opportunistic infection

REFERENCES

1. Centers for Disease Control and Prevention. 1993 revised classification system for HIV infection and expanded surveillance case definition for AIDS among adolescents and adults. *MMWR–Morbidity & Mortality Weekly Report.* 41(RR-17):1-19, 1992 Dec 18.

2. McDougal JS, Kennedy MS, Sligh JM, Cort SP, Mawle A, Nicholson JK. Binding of the HTLV-III/LAV to T4+ T cells by a complex of the 110K molecule and the T4 molecule. *Science.* 231:382-385, 1985.

3. Moss AR, Bacchetti P. Natural history of HIV infection. *AIDS.* 3:55-61, 1989.

4. Rutherford GW, Lifson AR, Hessol NA, Darrow WW, O'Malley PM, Buchbinder SP, Barnhart JL, Bodecker TW, Cannon L, Doll LS, et al. Course of

HIV-1 in a cohort of homosexual and bisexual men: An 11-year follow-up study. *British Medical Journal.* 301:1183-1188, 1990.

5. Munoz A, Wang MC, Bass S, Taylor JM, Kingsley LA, Chmiel JS, Polk BF. Acquired immunodeficiency syndrome (AIDS)–free time after human immunodeficiency virus type 1 (HIV-1) seroconversion in homosexual men. *American Journal of Epidemiology.* 130:530-539, 1989.

6. Rezza G, Lazzarin A, Angarano G, Sinicco A, Pristera R, Ortona L, Barbanera M, Gafa S, Tirelli U, Salassa B, et al. The natural history of HIV infection in intravenous drug users: Risk of disease progression in a cohort of seroconverters. *AIDS.* 3:87-90, 1989.

7. Selwyn PA, Hartel D, Schoenbaum EE, Davenny K. Rates and predictors of progression to HIV disease and AIDS in a cohort of intravenous drug users (IVDUs), 1985-1990. (Abstract F.C.111.) *International Conference on AIDS, San Francisco, CA, June 22, 1990*;2:117.

8. Medley GF, Anderson RM, Cox DR, Billard L. Incubation period of AIDS in patients infected via blood transfusion. *Nature.* 328:719-721, 1987.

9. Ward JW, Bush TJ, Perkins HA, Lieb LE, Allen JR, Goldfinger D, Samson SM, Pepkowite SH, Fernando LP, Holland PV, et al. The natural history of transfusion-associated infection with human immunodeficiency virus. *New England Journal of Medicine.* 321:947-952, 1989.

10. Goedert JJ, Kessler CM, Aledort LM, Biggar RJ, Andes WA, White GC 2nd, Drummond JE, Vaidya K, Mann DL, Eyster ME, et al. A prospective study of human immunodeficiency virus type 1 infection and the development of AIDS in subjects with hemophilia. *New England Journal of Medicine.* 321:1141-1148, 1989.

11. Auger I, Thomas P, De Gruttola V, Morse D, Moore D, Williams R, Truman B, Lawrence CE. Incubation periods for paediatric AIDS patients. *Nature.* 336:575-577, 1988.

12. Krasinski K, Borkowsky W, Holzman RS. Prognosis of human immunodeficiency virus in children and adolescents. *Pediatric Infectious Disease Journal.* 8:216-220, 1989.

13. Goedert JJ, Biggar RJ, Melbye M, Mann DL, Wilson S, Gail MH, Grossman AJ, DeGioia RA, Sanchez LX, Weiss SH, et al. Effect of T4 count and cofactors on the incidence of AIDS in homosexual men infected with human immunodeficiency virus. *JAMA.* 257:331-334, 1987.

14. Nicholson JKA, Spira TJ, Aloisio CH, Jones BM, Kennedy MS, Holman RC, McDougal JS. Serial determinations of HIV-1 titers in HIV-infected homosexual men: Association of rising titers with CD4 T cell depletion and progression to AIDS. *AIDS Research and Human Retroviruses.* 5:205-215, 1989.

15. Lang W, Perkins H, Anderson RE, Royce R, Jewell N, Windelstein W. Patterns of T-lymphocyte changes with human immunodeficiency virus infection: From seroconversion to the development of AIDS. *Journal of Acquired Immune Deficiency Syndrome.* 2:63-69, 1989.

16. Lange MA, de Wolf F, Goudsmit J. Markers for progression of HIV infection. *AIDS.* 3(Suppl 1):S153-160, 1989.

17. Taylor JM, Fahey JL, Detels R, Giorgi J. CD4 percentage, CD4 numbers, and CD4:CD 8 ratio in HIV infection: Which to choose and how to use. *Journal of Acquired Immune Deficiency Syndrome*. 2:114-124, 1989.

18. Masur H, Ognibene FP, Yarchoan R, Shelhamer JH, Baird BF, Travis W, Suffredini AF, Deyton L, Kovacs JA, Falloon J, et al. CD4 counts as predictors of opportunistic pneumonias in human immunodeficiency virus (HIV) infection. *Annals of Internal Medicine*. 111:223-231, 1989.

19. Fahey JL, Taylor JMG, Detels R., Hofmann B, Melmed R, Mishanian P, Giorgi JV, et al. The prognostic value of cellular and serologic markers in infection with human immunodeficiency virus type 1. *New England Journal of Medicine*. 322:166-172, 1990.

20. Fernandez-Cruz E, Desco M, Garcia Montes M, Longo N, Gonzalez B, Zabay JM. Immunological and serological markers predictive of progression to AIDS in a cohort of HIV-infected drug users. *AIDS*. 4:987-994, 1990.

21. National Institutes of Health. State-of-the-art conference on azidothymidine therapy for early HIV infection. *American Journal of Medicine*. 89:335-344, 1990.

22. CDC. Guidelines for prophylaxis against *Pneumocystis carinii* pneumonia for persons infected with human immunodeficiency virus. *MMWR–Morbidity & Mortality Weekly Report*. 41(No. RR-4):1-11, 1992.

23. Fischl MA, Richman DD, Hansen N, Collier AC, Carey JT, Para MF, Hardy WD, Dolin R, Powderly WG, Allan JD, et al. The safety and efficacy of zidovudine (AZT) in the treatment of subjects with mildly symptomatic human immunodeficiency virus type 1 (HIV) infection: A double blind, placebo controlled trial. *Annals of Internal Medicine*. 112:727-737, 1990.

24. Volberding PA, Lagakos SW, Koch MA, Pettinelli C, Myers MW, Booth DK, Balfour HH Jr, Reichman AC, Bartlett JA, Hirsch MS, et al. Zidovudine in asymptomatic human immunodeficiency virus infection: A controlled trial in persons with fewer than 500 CD4-positive cells per cubic millimeter. *New England Journal of Medicine*. 322:941, 1990.

25. Lagakos S, Fischl MA, Stein DS, Lim L, Volberding PA. Effects of zidovudine therapy in minority and other subpopulations with early HIV infection. *JAMA*. 266:2709-2712, 1991.

26. Easterbrook PJ, Keruly JC, Creagh-Kirk T, Richman DD, Chaisson RE, Moore RD. Racial and ethnic differences in outcome in zidovudine-treated patients with advanced HIV disease. *JAMA*. 266:2713-2718, 1991.

27. Hamilton JD, Hartigan PM, Simberkoff MS, Day PL, Diamond GA, Dickinson GM, Drusano GL, Egonin MJ, George WL, Gordin FM, et al. A controlled trial of early versus late treatment with zidovudine in symptomatic human immunodeficiency virus infection. *New England Journal of Medicine*. 326:437-443, 1992.

28. CDC. Classification system for human T-lymphotropic virus type III/lymphadenopathy-associated virus infections. *MMWR–Morbidity & Mortality Weekly Report*. 35:334-339, 1986.

29. National Institutes of Health. State-of-the-art conference on azidothymidine therapy for early HIV infection. *American Journal of Medicine*. 39:335-344, 1990 .

30. CDC. Guidelines for prophylaxis against *Pneumocystis carinii* pneumonia for persons infected with human immunodeficiency virus. *MMWR–Morbidity & Mortality Weekly Report*. 41(RR-4):1-11, 1992.

31. Fishl MA, Richman DD, Hansen N, Collier AC, Covey JT, Pasa MF, Hardy WD, Dolin R, Powderly WG, Allan JD, et al. The safety and efficacy of zidovudine (AZT) in the treatment of subjects with mildly symptomatic human immunodeficiency virus type 1 (HIV) infection: A double blind, placebo controlled trial. *Annals of Internal Medicine*. 112:727-737, 1990.

32. Volberding PA, Lagakos SW, Koch MA, Pettinelli C, Myers MW, Booth DK, Balfour HH Jr, Reichman RC, Bartlett JA, Hirsch MS, et al. Zidovudine in asymptomatic human immunodeficiency virus infection: A controlled trial in persons with fewer than 500 CD 4-positive cells per cubic millimeter. *New England Journal of Medicine*. 322:941, 1990.

33. Lagakos S, Fischl MA, Stein DS, Lim L, Volberding PA. Effects of zidovudine therapy in minority and other subpopulations with early HIV infection. *JAMA*. 266:2709-2712, 1991.

34. Easterbrook PJ, Keruly JC, Creagh-Kirk T, Richman DD, Chaisson RE, Moore RD. Racial and ethnic differences in outcome in zidovudine-treated patients with advanced HIV disease. *JAMA*. 266:2713-2718, 1991.

35. Hamilton JD, Hartigan PM, Simberkoff MS, Day PL, Diamond GA, Dickinson GM, Drusano GL, Egonin MJ, George WL, Gordin FM, et al. A controlled trial of early versus late treatment with zidovudine in symptomatic human immunodeficiency virus infection. *New England Journal of Medicine*. 326:437-443, 1992.

36. National Institutes of Health. State-of-the-art conference on azidothymidine therapy for early HIV infection. *American Journal of Medicine*. 89:335-344, 1990.

37. CDC. Classification system for human immunodeficiency virus (HIV) infection in children under 13 years of age. *MMWR–Morbidity & Mortality Weekly Report*. 36(15):225-230, 235-236, 1987 Apr 24.

38. CDC. Update: Acquired immunodeficiency syndrome (AIDS)–United States. *MMWR–Morbidity & Mortality Weekly Report*. 32:688-691, 1984.

39. CDC. Revision of the case definition of acquired immunodeficiency syndrome for national reporting–United States. *MMWR–Morbidity & Mortality Weekly Report*. 34:373-375, 1985.

40. CDC. Classification system for human T-lymphotropic virus type III/lymphadenopathy-associated virus infections. *MMWR–Morbidity & Mortality Weekly Report*. 35:334-339, 1986.

41. Redfield RR, Wright DC, Tramont ED. The Walter Reed staging classification for HTLV-III/LAV infection. *New England Journal of Medicine*. 314(2):131-132, 1986 Jan 9.

42. Haverkos HW, Gottlieb MS, Killen JY, Edelman R. Classification of HTLV-III/LAV-related diseases. [Letter.] *Journal of Infectious Diseases.* 152:1095, 1985.

43. Pahwa S, Kaplan M, Fikrig S, Sarngadharan MG, Popovic M, Gallo RC. Spectrum of human T-cell lymphotropic virus type III infection in children. *JAMA*. 255:2299-2305, 1986.

44. Scott GB, Anisman L, Zaldivar ML, Parks WP. Natural history of HTLV-III/LAV infections in children. Presented at the International Conference on AIDS, Paris, June 1986.

45. Ward JW, Grindon AJ, Feorino PM, Schable C, Parvin M, Allen JR. Laboratory and epidemiologic evaluation of an enzyme immunoassay for antibodies to HTLV-III. *JAMA*. 256:357-361, 1986.

46. Peterman TA, Jaffe, HW, Feorino PM, Getchell JP, Warfield DT, Haverkos HW, Stoneburner RL, Curran JW. Transfusion-associated acquired immunodeficiency syndrome in the United States. *JAMA*. 254:2913-2917, 1985.

47. Jaffe HW, Feorino PM, Darrow WW, O'Malley PM, Getchell JP, Warfield DT, Jones BM, Echenberg DF, Francis DP, Curran JW. Persistent infection with human T-lymphotropic virus type III/lymphotropic-associated virus in apparently healthy homosexual men. *Annals of Internal Medicine*. 102:627-628, 1985.

48. CDC. Update: acquired immunodeficiency syndrome (AIDS)–United States. *MMWR–Morbidity & Mortality Weekly Report*. 32:688-691, 1984.

49. CDC. Revision of the case definition of acquired immunodeficiency syndrome for national reporting–United States. *MMWR–Morbidity & Mortality Weekly Report*. 34:373-375, 1985.

50. CDC. Update: Acquired immunodeficiency syndrome (AIDS)–United States. *MMWR–Morbidity & Mortality Weekly Report*. 32:688-691, 1984.

51. CDC. Revision of the case definition of acquired immunodeficiency syndrome for national reporting–United States. *MMWR–Morbidity & Mortality Weekly Report*. 34:373-375, 1985.

52. CDC. Classification system for human T-lymphotropic virus type III/lymphadenopathy-associated virus infections. *MMWR–Morbidity & Mortality Weekly Report*. 35:334-339, 1986.

53. CDC. Recommendations for assisting in the prevention of perinatal transmission of human T-lymphotropic virus type III/lymphadenopathy-associated virus and acquired immunodeficiency syndrome. *MMWR–Morbidity & Mortality Weekly Report*. 34:721-6, 731-732, 1985.

54. CDC. Additional recommendations to reduce sexual and drug abuse-related transmission of human T-lymphotropic virus type III/lymphadenopathy-associated virus. *MMWR–Morbidity & Mortality Weekly Report*. 35:152-155, 1986.

55. CDC. Classification system for human T-lymphotropic virus type III/lymphadenopathy-associated virus infections. *MMWR–Morbidity & Mortality Weekly Report*. 35(20):334-339, 1986 May 23.

56. Gallo RC, Salahuddin SZ, Popovic M, Shearer GM, Kaplan M, Haynes BF, Palker TJ, Redfield R, Oleska J, Safai B, et al. Frequent detection and isolation of

cytopathic retroviruses (HTLV-III) from patients with AIDS and at risk for AIDS. *Science*. 224:500-503, 1984.

57. Barre-Sinoussi F, Chermann JC, Rey F, Mugeyre MT, Chamaret S, Gruest J, Dauguet C, Axler-Blin C, Vezinet-Brun F, Rouzioux C, Rozenbaum W, Montagnier L. Isolation of a T-lymphotropic retrovirus from a patient at risk for acquired immune deficiency syndrome (AIDS). *Science*. 220:868-871, 1983.

58. Levy JA, Hoffman AD, Kramer SM, Landis JA, Shimabukuro JM, Oshiro LS. Isolation of hymphocytopathic retroviruses from San Francisco patients with AIDS. *Science*. 225:840-842, 1984.

59. Coffin J, Haase A, Levy JA, Montagnier L, Oroszlan S, Teich N, Temin H, Toyoshima K, Varmas H, Vogt P, et al. Human immunodeficiency viruses. [Letter.] *Science*. 232:697, 1986.

60. CDC. Revision of the case definition of acquired immunodeficiency syndrome for national reporting–United States. *MMWR–Morbidity & Mortality Weekly Report*. 34:373-375, 1985.

61. Haverkos HW, Gottlieb MS, Killen JY, Eldelman R. Classification of HTLV-III/LAC-related diseases. [Letter.] *Journal of Infectious Diseases*. 152:1095, 1985.

62. Redfield RR, Wright DC, Tramont EC. The Walter Reed staging classification for HTLV-III/LAV infection. *New England Journal of Medicine*. 314:131-132, 1986.

63. CDC. Antibodies to a retrovirus etiologically associated with acquired immunodeficiency syndrome (AIDS) in populations with increased incidences of the syndrome. *MMWR–Morbidity & Mortality Weekly Report*. 33:377-379, 1984.

64. CDC. Update: public health service workshop on human T-lymphotropic virus type III antibody testing–United States. *MMWR–Morbidity & Mortality Weekly Report*. 34:477-478, 1985.

65. CDC. Additional recommendations to reduce sexual and drug abuse-related transmission of human T-lymphotropic virus type III/lymphadenopathy-associated virus. *MMWR–Morbidity & Mortality Weekly Report*. 35:152-155, 1986.

66. Selik RM, Haverkos HW, Curran JW. Acquired immune deficiency syndrome (AIDS) trends in the United States, 1978-1982. *American Journal of Medicine*. 76:493-500, 1984.

67. Sarngadharan MG, Popovic M, Bruch L, Schupbach J, Gallo RC. Antibodies reactive with human T-lymphotropic retroviruses (HTLV-III) in the serum of patients with AIDS. *Science*. 224:506-508, 1984.

68. Safai B, Sarngadharan MG, Groopman JE, Arnett K, Popovic M, Sliski A, Schupbach J, Gallo RC. Seroepidemiological studies of human T-lymphotropic retrovirus type III in acquired immunodeficiency syndrome. *Lancet*. I:1438-1440, 1984.

69. Laurence J, Brun-Vezinet F, Schutzer SE, Rouzioux C, Klatzmann D, Barre-Sinoussi F, Chermann JC, Montagnier L. Lymphadenopathy associated viral antibody in AIDS. Immune correlations and definition of a carrier state. *New England Journal of Medicine*. 311:1269-1273, 1984.

70. Sarngadharan MG, Popovic M, Bruch L, Schupbach J, Gallo RC. Antibodies reactive with human T-lymphotropic retroviruses (HTLV-III) in the serum of patients with AIDS. *Science.* 224:506-508, 1984.

71. Safai B, Sarngadharan MG, Groopman JE, Arnett K, Popovic M, Sliski A, Schupbach J, Gallo AC. Seroepidemiological studies of human T-lymphotropic retrovirus type III in acquired immunodeficiency syndrome. *Lancet.* I:1438-1440, 1984.

72. Laurence J, Brun-Vezinet F, Schutzer SE, Rouzioux C, Klatzmann D, Barre-Sinoussi F, Chermann JC, Montagnier L. Lymphadenopathy associated viral antibody in AIDS. Immune correlations and definition of a carrier state. *New England Journal of Medicine.* 311:1269-1273, 1984.

73. Ho DD, Sarngadharan MG, Resnick L, Dimarzo-Vernese F, Rota TR, Hirsch MS. Primary human T-lymphotropic virus type III infection. *Annals of Internal Medicine.* 103:880-883, 1985.

74. Cooper DA, Gold J, Maclean P, Donovan B, Finlayson R, Barnes TG, Michelmore HM, Brooke P, Penug R. Acute AIDS retrovirus infection. Definition of a clinical illness associated with seroconversion. *Lancet.* I:537-540, 1985.

75. Haverkos HW, Gottlieb MS, Killen JY, Eldelman R. Classification of HTLV-III/LAV-related diseases. [Letter.] *Journal of Infectious Diseases.* 152:1095, 1985.

76. Redfield RR, Wright DC, Tramont EC. The Walter Reed staging classification for HTLV-III/LAV infection. *New England Journal of Medicine.* 314(2):131-132, 1986 Jan 9.

77. Ibid.

Appendix C

Internet Resource Sites

This appendix contains examples of Internet sites relevant to HIV and AIDS. This should not be construed as a comprehensive list of Internet resources; rather it is intended to provide samples of the types of information available via the Internet. In addition, it is important to remember that the addresses–or Universal Resource Locators (URLs)–for gopher and World Wide Web sites often change.

DISCUSSION LISTS

Caregivers Support
  caregivers@queernet.org
HIV-SUPPORT
  hiv-support@web-depot.com
Physicians' and Psychotherapists' Resource
  HIV-Docs@web-depot.com

USENET NEWSGROUPS

CLARI.TW.HEALTH.AIDS
MISC.HEALTH.AIDS
SCI.MED.AIDS

GOPHER SITES

AIDS Book Review Journal
gopher://ucsbuxa.ucsb.edu:3001/11/.Journals/.A/.AIDS
CDC National AIDS Clearinghouse Gopher
gopher://cdcnac.aspensys.com:72/11/
HIVNET
gopher://hivnet.org
NIH AIDS-related Gopher
gopher://odie.niaid.nih.gov/11/aids

WORLD WIDE WEB SITES

AIDS Pathology (University of Utah)
http://www-medlib.med.utah.edu/WebPath/AIDS.html
AIDS Virtual Library
http://www.actwin.com/aids/vl.html
Alternative Medicine
http://www.pitt.edu/~cbw/altm.html
Australian HIV Electronic Media Information Review
http://florey.biosci.uq.oz.au/hiv/HIV_EMIR.html
Canadian HIV Trials Network
http://unixg.ubc.ca:780/~fortin/Marcel.html
Center for AIDS Prevention Studies
http://chanane.ucsf.edu/capsweb/index.html
Condom Country
http://www.ag.com/condom/country
DeathNET
http://www.islandnet.com/~deathnet
HIV Database–Los Alamos National Laboratory
http://hiv-web.lanl.gov/
Kairos Support for Caregivers
http://www.catalog.com/kairos/welcome.htm

Medscape's AIDS Page
http://www.medscape.com/Home/Medscape-AIDS/Medscape-AIDS.html
National Centre in HIV Social Research (Australia)
http://www.bhs.mq.au/nchsr.html
Positive Approaches to HIV and AIDS (United Kingdom)
http://phymat.bham.ac.uk/LGB/positive.html
The Information Exchange
http://www.dircon.co.uk/blue/star/:xhome.htm
The Red Ribbon Net
http://worldclass.com/redribbn/
The Safer Sex Page
http://www.cmpharm.ucsf.edu/~troyer/safesex.html
The TB/HIV Research Laboratory
http://www.brown.edu/Research/TB-HIV_Lab/
United Kingdom Clinical Trials
http://www.dircon.co.uk/blue/star/:xa2z.htm
WHO Global Programme on AIDS
http://gpawww.who.ch/gpahome.htm

Appendix D

Organization Information

This appendix contains the names, addresses, and telephone numbers for organizations and institutions referred to throughout the text. Entries are arranged alphabetically by organization name.

Agency for Health Care Policy and Research
Department of Health and Human Services
Public Health Service
Executive Office Center
2101 E. Jefferson Street
Rockville, MD 20852
(301) 594-8364

AIDS Clinical Trials Information Service (ACTIS)
P.O. Box 6421
Rockville, MD 20850
(800) TRIALS-A

AIDS Information Center
Library Service (142D)
VA Medical Center
4150 Clement Street
San Francisco, CA 94121
(415) 221-4810 ext. 3305

AIDS Information Exchange Resource Centre
African Regional Health Education Centre
Department of Preventive and Social Medicine
University of Ibadan
Ibadan, Nigeria

AIDS Information Network
32 N. 3rd Street
Philadelphia, PA 19106
(215) 922-5120

AIDS Program
Department of Medicine
San Francisco General Hospital
Building 80
Ward 84
1001 Potrero Avenue
San Francisco, CA 94110
(415) 206-8410

AIDS Resource Center (Dallas)
2701 Reagan
Dallas, TX 75219
(214) 521-5124

AIDS Social History Programme
Department of Public Health and Policy
London School of Hygiene and Tropical Medicine
Bureau of Hygiene and Tropical Diseases
Keppel Street
London, WC1E 7HT, England

AIDS Treatment Information Service (ATIS)
P.O. Box 6303
Rockville, MD 20848-6003
(800) HIV-0440
(800) 243-7012 (Deaf access)
(301) 735-6616 (Fax)

CD Resources, Inc.
118 W. 74th Street
Suite 2A
New York, NY 10023
(212) 580-2263

Centers for Disease Control and Prevention (CDC)
Department of Health and Human Services
Public Health Service
1600 Clifton Road, N.E.
Atlanta, GA 30333
(404) 639-3286

Department of Health and Human Services
200 Independence Avenue, S.W.
Washington, DC 20201
(202) 619-0257

Federal Centre for AIDS
Department of National Health and Welfare
301 Elgin Street
Ottawa, Ontario
KlA OL2
Canada

Food and Drug Administration
Department of Health and Human Services
Public Health Service
5600 Fishers Lane
Rockville, MD 20857

Gay Men's Health Crisis (GMHC)
129 W. 20th Street
New York, NY 10011
(212) 807-7035
(212) 807-7517

Global Programme on AIDS
World Health Organization
20 Avenue Appia
CH-1211
Geneva 27, Switzerland
(+4122) 791.37.70

Health Resources and Services Administration (HRSA)
Department of Health and Human Services
Public Health Service
5600 Fishers Lane
Rockville, MD 20857
(301) 443-6745

Indian Health Service
Department of Health and Human Services
Public Health Service
Parklawn Building
5600 Fishers Lane
Rockville, MD 20857
(301) 443-3593

Los Angeles Gay and Lesbian Community Services Center
1213 N. Highland Avenue
Los Angeles, CA 90028
(213) 993-7415

National AIDS Clearinghouse (NAC)
P.O. Box 6003
1600 Research Boulevard
Rockville, MD 20850
(800) 458-5231

National AIDS Hotline
(800) 342-AIDS
(800) 342-SIDA (Spanish access)
(800) AIDS-TTY (Deaf access)

National Institute of Allergy and Infectious Diseases (NIAID)
NIH Building 31
9000 Rockville Pike
Bethesda, MD 20205
(301) 496-5717

National Institutes of Health (NIH)
Department of Health and Human Services
Public Health Service
9000 Rockville Pike
Bethesda, MD 20892
(301) 496-4000

National Library of Medicine (NLM)
8600 Rockville Pike
Bethesda, MD 20209
(800) 638-8480

New York Public Library
5th Avenue and 42nd Street
New York, NY 10016-0109
(212) 930-0831

Norman Public Library
225 N. Webster
Norman, OK 73069
(405) 321-1481

Paramount Publishing
P.O. Box 5630
Norwalk, CT 06856
(203) 838-4400

Pasteur Institute
35-38 Rue du Doctor Roux
75015 Paris, France

Project Inform
347 Dolores Street
Suite 301
San Francisco, CA 94110
(800) 822-7422
(800) 334-7422 (California only)

Public Health Service (PHS)
Parklawn Building
5600 Fishers Lane
Rockville, MD 20856
(301) 443-2414

San Francisco AIDS Foundation
333 Valencia Street
4th Floor
San Francisco, CA 94103
(415) 864-4376

Southeast Florida AIDS Information Network
Louis Calder Memorial Library
University of Miami School of Medicine
P.O. Box 016950
Miami, FL 33101

Substance Abuse and Mental Health Services Administration (SAMHSA)
Department of Health and Human Services
Public Health Service
Parklawn Building
5600 Fishers Lane
Rockville, MD 20857

Walter Reed Army Institute of Research
6825 16th Street, N.W.
Washington, DC 20307-5100

Index